The Caring Imperative in Education

The Caring Imperative in Education

Madeleine Leininger and Jean Watson, Editors

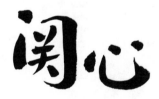

关心

CARING
关: PASSAGE
TO THE
心: HEART

Center for Human Caring

National League for Nursing
Pub. No. 41-2308

Copyright © 1990
National League for Nursing
350 Hudson Street, New York, NY 10014

ISBN 0-88737-470-0

The views expressed in this publication represent the views of the authors and do not necessarily reflect the official views of the National League for Nursing.

This book was set in Baskerville by Publications Development Company. The editor and designer was Allan Graubard. St. Mary's Press was the printer and binder.

The cover was designed by Lillian Welsh.

Printed in the United States of America

Contents

Contributors

Cathy Appleton, RN, is Assistant Professor, Florida Atlantic University, Boca Raton, Florida, and PhD student, University of Colorado Health Sciences Center, School of Nursing, Denver, Colorado.

Janet A. Bauer, PhD, RN, is Assistant Professor, Cedarville College, Cedarville, Ohio.

Anne H. Bishop, EdD, MSN, BSN, RN, is Professor of Nursing, Lynchburg College, Lynchburg, Virginia.

Anne Boykin, PhD, RN, is Director, Division of Nursing, Florida Atlantic University, Boca Raton, Florida.

Mary Woods Byrne, PhD, RN, is Chairperson, Undergraduate Nursing Program, College of Mount Saint Vincent, Riverdale, New York.

Christina L. S. Evans, MSN, CNA, RN, is a Specialist, Nursing Administration, Kingswood Hospital, Ferndale, Michigan.

Rauda Gelazis, MNEd, RN, is Associate Professor, Ursuline College, Pepper Pile, Ohio, and PhD student, Wayne State University School of Nursing, Detroit, Michigan.

Diana Gendron, MS, BS, is Senior Tutor, Faculty of Nursing, University of Toronto, Toronto, Ontario.

Maxine Greene, PhD, is Professor, Teachers College, Columbia University, New York, New York.

Judith Haber, PhD, RN, CS, is Director, Department of Nursing, College of Mount Saint Vincent, Riverdale, New York.

Mary Hagedorn, MS, RN, CNS, is a PhD student at the University of Colorado School of Nursing, Boulder, Colorado.

Sigríður Halldórsdóttir, MSN, RN, is Assistant Professor, University of Iceland, Reykjavík, Iceland.

Sonya Hardin, MSN, RN, is a PhD candidate at the University of Colorado Health Sciences Center, Denver, Colorado.

Nancy Klenk Hill, PhD, is Associate Professor of Humanities, University of Colorado/Boulder, Boulder, Colorado.

Mark Klimek, MSN, RN, is Assistant Professor of Nursing, Cedarville College, Cedarville, Ohio, and PhD student, Wayne State University, Detroit, Michigan.

Dixie Koldjeski, PhD, RN, FAAN, is the former Interim Director, Doctoral Program, University of Pittsburgh School of Nursing, Pittsburgh, Pennsylvania.

Silvia Prodan Lange, MN, RN, CS, is Clinical Specialist in Psychiatric/ Mental Health Nursing, Pacific Presbyterian Medical Center, San Francisco, California.

Cheryl Demerath Learn, MS, RN, BSN, is Lecturer, University of New Mexico, Albuquerque, New Mexico and PhD student at the University of Colorado, School of Nursing, Denver, Colorado.

Reinhold P. Marxhausen, BFA, Professor of Art, Concordia Teachers College, Seward, Nebraska.

Sharie Metcalfe, MS, BS, RN, is a PhD student at Wayne State University, Detroit, Michigan.

Barbara Krainovich Miller, EdD, RN, is Chairperson, Graduate Nursing Program, College of Mount Saint Vincent, Riverdale, New York.

Patricia Moccia, PhD, RN, is Vice President, Division of Education and Accreditation Services, National League for Nursing.

Tommie P. Nelms, PhD, RD, is Assistant Professor at Georgia State University, Atlanta, Georgia.

Nancy A. O'Connor, MSN, RNC, is a Certified Adult Nurse Practitioner, and a PhD student, Wayne State University, Detroit, Michigan.

Linda J. Postlethwaite, RN, is an MSN candidate, Florida Atlantic University, Division of Nursing, Boca Raton, Florida.

John R. Scudder, Jr., EdD, MA, BA, is Professor of Philosophy, Lynchburg College, Lynchburg, Virginia.

Mary Lou Sheston, MSN, RN, is Assistant Professor, Thomas Jefferson University, Philadelphia, Pennsylvania.

Mary Ellen Symanski, MS, RN, is Assistant Professor of Nursing, University of Maine, Orono, Maine, and PhD student, Wayne State University, Detroit, Michigan.

Preface

This work is an official publication of the University of Colorado Center for Human Caring in collaboration with the International Association for Human Caring. It is an outgrowth of the 11th National/International Caring Conference held in Denver, Colorado, April 30–May 2, 1989.

The Center for Human Caring is exploring new ways to advance the art and science of human caring in education, research, and practice. The think tank efforts in the center range from academic curricular and health policy activities to developing new philosophies, theories, ethics, and methods associated with knowledge of caring. This work includes developing demonstration projects for teaching, studying, and practicing traditional and new clinical caring and healing modalities.

The central purpose of the International Association for Human Caring is to serve as a scholarly forum for nurses to advance knowledge of care and caring within the discipline of nursing. Its goals are to (1) identify major philosophical, epistemological, and professional dimensions of care and caring to advance the body of knowledge that constitutes nursing and to help other disciplines use care and caring knowledge in human relationships; (2) explicate the nature, scope, and functions of care and caring and its relationship to nursing; (3) identify the major components, processes, and patterns of care and caring in relationship to nursing; (4) stimulate nurse scholars internationally to systematically investigate care and caring and to share findings with colleagues; and (5) share knowledge through publication and public forum.

The conference, "The Caring Imperative in Education," was the first international conference for the Center and the 11th Caring Conference in the United States. It attracted professionals from seven different countries, with international presentations from Canada, Iceland, and Sweden. It was the first conference of its kind in helping to elucidate the issues, conflicts, and challenges associated with integration of the humanities and the aesthetic experience of caring in education. The conference theme was anchored by an opening session on the Aesthetics of Caring which was conveyed through visual and sound art presentations by Reinhold Marxhausen; poetry on caring by Marilyn Krysl; and the creative literary and metaphorical scholarship of Professor Nancy Hill.

The distinguished keynote speakers, Professor Maxine Greene of Columbia Teachers College, and Dr. Patricia Moccia, Vice President of Education and Accreditation, National League for Nursing, introduced a liberalizing humanities framework for caring in education and concluded with a political call to consciousness—to choose to care. Other topics included the tensions and passions of caring; the teaching and practice of caring in academe and administration. Finally, the conference focused on deciding to care, as a way of developing knowledge of caring, that underpins and affects all educational processes and politics.

These keynote speakers, invited presenters, combined with progressive scientific studies and global caring perspectives, contributed to diverse, yet comprehensive approaches to the imperative of caring in education. The broad aim for suggesting the caring imperative was to evoke integrative, liberalizing, and freeing behavior, and education for the whole person.

At the same time, we have to realize that education is finally and ultimately a human experience and human act for which there can be no final agreements or answers. Perhaps it is the passion and commitment to the caring imperative in education and in health care that can shape the dialogue and the dialectic, frame the issues, and make a new clearing—a clearing whereby caring can be kept alive and space for new possibilities can emerge for teachers and students and systems alike. This conference publication on the caring imperative in education is only one of many clearings that need to be made if we are to educate, liberalize, and free ourselves; if we are to reclaim the beauty and aesthetics of wholeness; if we are to restore and preserve the art and science of human caring and healing for ourselves and society at large.

My thanks and continuing appreciation go to the National League for Nursing for being a partner with the Center for Human Caring and in helping to create continuous clearings for other new possibilities by agreeing to be the official publication outlet for Center for Human Caring projects and activities.

Jean Watson, PhD, RN, FAAN
Professor of Nursing
Director, Center for Human Caring
University of Colorado
Health Sciences Center
Denver, Colorado

Conference Commentary

Coordinating the 1989 Caring Conference provided a unique and privileged perspective from which to consider the relationship between caring and education. An early task was to choose a conference title. The Caring Imperative in Education captured the commitment of the International Association for Human Caring Board to the importance of the topic. The appeal of this title became apparent as potential speakers were contacted and abstracts submitted. Two broad themes emerged—education *about* caring and caring *in* the educational process. The integration of perspectives from the arts and humanities brought emphasis to the concepts that most forcefully unite education and caring. These concepts are the dignity of the individual person and freedom.

The 11th International Caring Conference offered many opportunities for participants to expand their perspectives regarding caring and education—to become more free and creative in their approaches to their own life commitments. Not everything presented pleased everyone. That's "o.k." (In fact, several of the conference participants, in their evaluation of the conference, indicated that the conference schedule itself was particularly "un-freeing." That aspect of the evaluations was communicated to future conference planners.)

In summary, I believe that the conference objectives were well met. I look forward, while reading the contributions to this collection of conference papers, to re-thinking many of the ideas that were presented, and to continue to grow as a care provider and educator. Finally, it was a true privilege to have a significant role in making this conference possible.

Ruth M. Neil, PhD, MN, RN
Coordinator 11th National / International Caring Conference

University of Colorado
School of Nursing
Denver, Colorado

Introduction

CARE: THE IMPERATIVE OF
NURSING EDUCATION AND SERVICE

More than three decades have passed since a few nurse scholars began to study the phenomenon of care in a systematic and rigorous way as the essence and distinct feature of nursing. This cultural care movement has been gaining momentum since 1980 as more nurses are now studying the humanistic clinical, historical, transcultural, and other diverse dimensions of human care and caring. It has captured the past interests and deeply valued posture of many nurses of the pre-World War II era, and it has stimulated the intellectual, theoretical, and research interests of this generation of nursing students. This cultural movement has reinforced my long-standing position and efforts to make care the central focus and essence of the discipline of nursing.

It is a most encouraging trend that today more nurses are studying the explicit meanings, expressions, patterns, and structure of care than ever before in nursing. These nurse scholars are discovering anew many of the largely hidden, covert, and "taken-for-granted" aspects of care in different life contexts from historical, epistemological, ontological, and transcultural nursing perspectives. These nurses are realizing that care can make a significant difference in healing, maintaining well-being, and in renewal of the nature of the human spirit. Human care is being studied with renewed vigor and enthusiasm to make care the hallmark of the discipline and profession of nursing.

1

One of the most encouraging developments is that faculty in schools of nursing are beginning to make care an imperative in teaching, research, and clinical-community practices. Care is becoming not only a desired philosophical and epistemological base of nursing knowledge, but also an ethical and moral imperative. In recent years, nursing faculty are deliberately beginning to use knowledge generated from care research. For example, nurses are drawing from nearly three decades of transcultural nursing research of Western and non-Western cultures with explicit care meanings and experiences. Other nursing knowledge is coming from philosophical questions about care; and others from direct clinical observations. Faculty are beginning to teach care concepts in-depth as related to the explicit meanings of comfort, enabling, presence, succorance, support, compassion, and nearly 85 other care constructs—concepts that have been limitedly known in their fullest meanings to nurses in the past. In addition, several theories about human care such as the theories of "Cultural Care Diversity and University" and "Self-Care," plus other theoretical perspectives are stimulating new lines of inquiry and generating valuable research findings that have been unknown in the nursing profession. These theoretical ideas and research findings are gradually entering the student-teacher learning context. It is also encouraging to find that students can differentiate between *generic* (lay) and *professional care,* and to value care meanings, symbols, and expressions of human care in caregiver and care-receiver situations.

Discovering similarities and differences among individuals, families and cultures worldwide has been another major achievement in education and clinical nursing practices. Teaching nursing students to be sensitive and responsive to transcultural care meanings, expressions, and needs has been one of the major developments in nursing curricula in this century, and it will be even more significant in the next one. There are, however, nurses who have not been exposed to existing explicit knowledge of care and care practices that have been generated during the past three decades. This body of care research knowledge and the philosophical treatises on human care and caring phenomena are important discoveries. There are also nurse clinicians and faculty who are still wed to teaching and practicing nursing from medical symptoms, diseased conditions, and treatments rather than focusing on human care as the essence of nursing. Moreover, there are nursing schools that have virtually no care content in their curricula except as linguistic care slogans or cliches. There are also some nursing service staff that eschew or devalue the importance of human care for medical treatments and technological tasks. Hence, there is much work yet to be done in nursing education and clinical practices to make human care a central, distinct, and imperative feature of nursing.

One should also realize that there are controversial positions about *if* and *how* human care is taught or learned. Some nurses contend that care is largely an "intuitive gift" and a "kind" or "benevolent attitude" which nurses are born with and use in their own unique ways. These nurses believe that care can not be taught nor learned. There are other nurses who hold care can only be taught by direct life experiences and human interactions. And, there are other nurses who have been studying and teaching care over an extended period of time, who hold that care can be explicitly taught using theoretical, research and clinical experiences with diverse teaching methods. These controversial teaching and learning postures are challenging nurses to rethink and reexamine care pedogical aspects in nursing education and practice.

With the growing cadre of care scholars, researchers, teachers, theoreticians, and clinicians gradually being committed to care, there is new hope and encouragement for generating much and unknown care knowledge. There is hope for nurses to build upon existing care knowledge to establish a firm care discipline and profession of nursing. There are indeed, nurses studying human care as a phenomenon for the first time in their professional work. There are also more positive attitudes about studying care than existed in the 1950's through the 1970's. I well remember that many nurse leaders during the 1980 era and after World War II often told me "You are wasting your time studying care as care is 'too feminine,' 'too soft,' 'too non-scientific,' and 'too vague.'" Moreover, they added that care could never be objectified, quantified, nor measurable, and, therefore could not be scientific. These nurse researchers were primarily interested in studying dramatic medical curses, performing technological tasks, and studying medical procedures and medical phenomenon. So, shifting nurses from a largely medical cure focus to a care focus was extremely difficult in those early days. It was also clear that care was not of central interest to many nurses. Care and caring was vaguely viewed an important factor to gain or regain health or to maintain well being. Gradually, these viewpoints began to change during the last few decades as a few care scholars and theoreticians remained firm and persistent in explicating care discoveries.

It is also important to note that there were two major developments in the 1970's that greatly stimulated nurses to value and study human care, and from broad and in-depth humanistic and scientific perspectives. The first was the Transcultural Nursing Society's annual conferences (beginning in 1974); the second was the National Research Care Conferences (beginning in 1978). Nurse leaders of these two national and international organizations held yearly open forums focused on care theory, research, and clinical practices. The conferences were highly stimulating and scholarly, and they were the only two continuous conferences in nursing focused on care for nearly two decades. It was encouraging and fascinating to gradually investigate different aspects of human care, and become excited about their discoveries. These nurses drew upon knowledge not only from nursing but from the social sciences, humanities, and many diverse sources to examine care phenomenon. The pioneering research work and thinking of Aamodt, Gaut, Gardner, Horn, Leininger, Ray, Larson, and Watson were some of the early and continuous leaders who struggled to study the humanistic, transcultural, and scientific aspects of care. Later, the thinking and care research of Reiman, Weiss, Benner, Gates, Luna, Wenger, Rosenbaum, McFarland, Valentine, Kauffman-Swanson and others added important findings and different knowledge and insights about human care and caring. Thus the two national nursing forums with multidisciplinary participants greatly advanced the discovery of care during the past two decades.

Since 1985, there have been a growing number of nurses interested in studying and writing about care. Care has become popular in nursing and in the public arena. With popularization of care, some nurses may not always search for the epistemic and historical work already done in nursing through research and critical study by the early care scholars. This early knowledge provides an essential base upon which to build, refine, and advance human care knowledge. Nonetheless, it is encouraging to see more nurses and especially nursing students become involved in the study of care. It is also promising for the profession that more nursing faculty and nursing service staff are becoming interested to study and use care concepts, principles, and research findings in their work. Faculty are beginning to learn about many different philosophical, theoretical, and creative ways to teaching and learning about care. They are also discovering some of the work by nursing care scholars, but also the thinking of poets, philosophers, artists, historians, ecologists, social scientists, educators, and others about humanistic and scientific care. These trends are helping to develop a collective consciousness about care and to institutionalize care in nursing education and service.

This book reflects some of the above trends and the extant thinking of scholars in nursing and other disciplines who are vitally interested in establishing human care as an imperative in nursing education and all human services. These ideas should stimulate nurses to reflect upon care from many different perspectives and world views. It should liberate nurses to think anew about the significance of human caring in all aspects of living, suffering, and dying. The contributors to this book are challenging the readers to think about new ways of teaching and learning about care and with a transcultural focus of all world cultures and human communities. Caring concepts, decisions, and actions must be fully studied to advance knowledge about human living, healing, and to maintain well-being in our present day world of violence and threats to the human spirit.

In sum, it is most encouraging to see nurses systematically studying the nature, epistemics, philosophic, and transcultural aspects of human care than ever before in the history of nursing. Care is becoming a central and major focus of nursing education and practice. In the future, I predict that this trend will continue and that care will become the major distinct and public contribution from the discipline of nursing. But much more systematic research and creative teaching–learning investigations on care are needed as well as to establish a public policy reality with rewards to nurses for their exquisite care contributions. Indeed, caring knowledge and practice must permeate our schools of nursing, universities, health centers, and world communities. Care with transcultural knowledge must become the arching framework for all aspects of nursing. The past covert or invisible aspects of human care by nurses must become known to all public consumers. When this occurs, nursing will be fully recognized and known as a profession and discipline with substantive knowledge base. These developments are a dream come true for me as an early and continuous care scholar and leader who has spearheaded, promoted, and remained an active researcher of human care for the past 40 years. It has indeed been a professional lifetime for me in advancing care as the essence of nursing, and as the powerful and distinctive attribute of the discipline.

Madeleine Leininger, PhD, RN, CTN, LHD, FAAN
Professor of Nursing and Anthropology
Wayne State University, Detroit, Michigan
President of the International Association of Human Caring

1

Serendipity

Reinhold P. Marxhausen

It should not be unusual that an artist has been asked to address an audience on the topic of caring, because it has to do with what we give our attention to. As a visual artist and a creative person, awareness of my surroundings and the people who live in it provides the source for my ideas and my art.

For everyone, as our surroundings become ordinary, it becomes more and more difficult to see anything that even relates to aesthetics in our lives. To go somewhere else to find beauty is only to run away from the extraordinary possibility that may exist in our ordinary lives.

I'm interested in perception and what we perceive as being ugly or beautiful. *Serendipity* means the possibility of making a happy chance discovery. I'm 67 years old; looking back, I can see that my life has been filled with serendipitous or fortuitous events. My stories may encourage you to consider and practice the insight and mindset that can lead to the magic transformation that can take place.

My first story, "Square Circle," is a true story about left-right brain activity. One morning, I opened my eyes and saw a spotlight over my bed. And this spotlight had a circular rainbow around its edge. To my left, the morning sun coming through the square window made this circle with a rainbow around it. I thought, "Fantastic!" In just a few minutes it disappeared. And I remembered it all day long; I felt good,

8 R. P. MARXHAUSEN

and I was singing, because I had this magic circle over my bed, and I didn't know where it came from.

It came back for several days. A part of me kept saying, "You ought to figure that out! There's no magic in life! That's impossible! How can light come through a square window and make a circle?" So part of me wanted to *know* where it came from, but part of me just liked it. That's how the left-right brain works; one part is poetic, and one is based on knowledge. I could feel the struggle of wanting to know and not wanting to know.

About the sixth day, I really wanted to know. I looked over to the right and on my wife's dresser was a vanity mirror with a beveled edge, and I thought, "Ah-ha. The light comes through the square window, goes over my bed, hits the mirror, and does the magic." And I got up out of bed, I went to the dresser, I turned the mirror to the wall, and I haven't seen the rainbow since.

I teach a course on creativity. This year, Halloween fell on the night that we had the night class. The class decided everyone should come to school in a costume. I decided that we would also go to the retirement home, and that each person would spend 30 or 45 minutes in a room with someone he or she didn't know. I asked the class how many wanted to do this, and not a single one wanted to. I said, "That's why we're doing it."

Everybody got dressed up so they could be anonymous and was assigned to a room. I gave them permission to hold hands and touch the people. Many of them told me that there was no conversation until the touching began. I'm sure it changed the lives of every one of my students.

Some years ago I worked with a surgeon in Lincoln, Nebraska, who had Alzheimer's disease. Typically, he had no memory, ran away from home, his wife shaved him every day, and he had no sense of self. I believe that each one of us is holistic, and just because the memory is gone doesn't mean that everything else is. I wanted to find this self that was Hiram. I did a series of exercises and projects; some worked, and some didn't. Since Hiram was a surgeon, he was good with scissors. We'd take magic markers and make some shapes, and he would cut those shapes out. He flinched when he nicked the magic marker lines. He was very precise, and he glued them down, and made collages.

Then I thought, "Well, he's a surgeon; he ought to know how to sew." I took an embroidery hoop, put a little piece of cloth across it, took a red magic marker, and put a stripe on the cloth. I showed him how to stitch. He was in the Army during World War II, and while he stitched the stripe, he wept, and talked about the bad things that happened. He did only several "sewing" projects, because they were too emotional for him.

We would also draw together; when I discovered small bits of writing in his drawings, I realized that he liked to write. I gave him blank pieces of paper and encouraged him to write, which he did. The scribbled writings were not readable, but he enjoyed the experience and felt very good. One day before I left the house with a handful of his writings, he pointed to them and said, "Those are mine." I said, "What did you say?" He said, "Those are mine." He didn't recognize his wife or his family or anybody, but those writings were real! Another day he sat there with a pencil and a blank piece of paper, and he asked, "How should I say this?" The question is: Are these writings by Hiram poetry, or are they not? I say they are. I call them "writing in tongues."

Some years ago I welded some wires to a doorknob as part of a sculpture. Out of curiosity, I put the knob to my ear; when I plucked the wires, I heard a beautiful sound. Since then, I've developed a musical toy that I call "stardust." They're made for the pocket and the hand, and they produce a wonderful sound, and my idea is that if everybody who takes drugs had one of these, we could eliminate the use of drugs and alcohol.

In a sculpture by Giacometti, the tall, gaunt bronze figures represent people. They look like old people, but these are like young people on drugs and alcohol who are bored and standing around saying, "What's happening, man?" They're just wondering when the parade will begin. Shakespeare said that all the world's a stage, and we are the actors on the stage; we make life interesting or we make life boring. And there's nothing more boring than a bored person, standing with his big feet on square one; he's arrogant, he thinks that he's right, that everybody else is wrong. Giacometti made this sculpture to identify a race of bored people. Many people I meet every day are just like that.

I like to wash dishes at home because it's when I get my best ideas. One night we had spaghetti, and I pulled the spaghetti strainer out of the dishwater and noticed that each hole held one drop of water. When I put my head inside the strainer, I noticed that each drop of water was magnifying the other drops. Then my question was, "How come each drop took a different picture?" So doing this boring job, I was thinking of physics and science. The next time we have spaghetti, I can look in the strainer and wonder.

On our back porch we have our white washer and dryer. One morning before I went to work I took a picture of the dryer. After another 100 photographs, in the morning, I realized that none were alike!

People say, "Nothing ever happens in my town; it's too small." Baloney! Wherever people live and where the sun shines, everything changes. North of the town where I live, there's a black sign with white letters. I drove by one day around sunset, and the white letters were black! Of course, I took a photograph. When I brought an enlargement to the bank, the people said, "Aren't the letters white?" I said, "Most of the time." It's your left brain that wants to know that the black paint is shiny and that it reflects the sunset; the white paint is dull, it absorbs light. Now your left brain is happy. But the magic is gone.

Somebody was watering the lawn at 9 p.m. I noticed that the house and the water had a golden color. As I rolled up the film in my camera, the sun set. I looked back as I went to the car, and all I saw was the wet house. Each day we miss many many moments that last only a minute. If we're not awake, then life is boring.

I had a table with a piece of tin on it. I didn't want the tin anymore, so I tore it off. Before I threw it away, I looked under the piece of tin where it stuck to the table, and I saw where the glue stuck to the tabletop. I framed it! This is part of my art collection, this piece of tin. After I'm gone, someone may try to decide what prompted me to do a painting of a tin table.

A man with a black car is parked downtown next to a yellow car. If he thinks his black car is always black, he's missing much of the excitement and change that are often different.

A snowplow in a little town in Nebraska is a wonderful piece of metal against the blue sky. Refugees from Manhattan or New York look at the art and ask, "What is all this supposed to mean?" If they don't see beauty in the snowplow in their town, they're certainly not going to see it in Manhattan. You've got to start where you live, and see and touch the flowers, and see the simple things. Then art becomes meaningful.

By saying "tomato," I conjure up an image that's round and red. One summer I found a tomato in my garden with a leg under it or something. This is a tomato. THIS is a tomato! See? These are all tomatoes! You know, I'm disrupting your preconceived ideas about tomatoes. If you don't eat tomatoes, they just die naturally in the garden. Until we realize tomatoes are not always red, we have this very limited view of what the world can be.

Driving to Omaha one day, in July, I saw a farmer had erected snow fences over the cows to keep them cool. It was noon and I was seeing zebras created by the shadows of fences. Last year in Wisner, Nebraska, I spoke to two hundred cattle farmers and their wives in a high school gym. I asked these farmers, "How many of you farmers would see these stripes on your cows if this was in your feedlot?" Not a single hand went up. Not a hand went up because they see cows! I don't know anything about cows but I see stripes! These examples show the difference between perception and looking.

My pictures of the side of a barn show a rusty nail right here in close-up and the side of a barn from a distance. Some of you can see the fish jumping out of the water or a little face or a flower. In California, in contrast, when the traffic stops and people are late for work and they're traveling 2 hours to get to work, and they're angry because of the traffic jams, they might have to learn how to use the right side of their brain and be able to look out of their cars and see the knots in the barn, or in the clouds, as we did when we were children. And we gave it up because we thought it was a childish thing to do. It's no longer childish to be able to have access to the resources open to each of us!

Ideas also help us to make connections. On the beach in California, I noticed that a baby pacifier and the kelp had the same color, the same shape, and the same texture as if they were brother and sister! Now, no one ever told me that! I found that out all by myself on the beach.

Sister Corita designed some designs for gas tanks in Boston because they were too plain. And people complained because they didn't understand what it meant. Last year I found a picture of the snow in the mountains in a *National Geographic Magazine*. And if Sister Corita were still living, she would be tickled pink to realize that somebody gave meaning to her abstraction, because she was just doing an abstraction. She was not doing mountain or snow. I'm the one who found the mountain and the snow.

In a painting by Mondrian, you can see the rectilinear images and lines and shapes, and a red shape in the bottom. I drove through a little town near Omaha recently, and I was surprised to find the same rectangles in a barbershop, with a little red bench in the same position. I've been teaching art for 35 years and the Mondrian image is in the back of my mind, you see. So when the day came, and the barbershop came, I could make the connection. The more information we amass, and the more problems we pile up on the back burner, when the magic, serendipitous moment, when the answer's there, we can make the connection, say "ah-ha! There it is! I've been waiting for you! Where have you been?"

If you fly a lot and look out of the windows you can see plowed fields over Kansas, Colorado, and Nebraska. They tore down an old building in Lincoln, Nebraska. I picked up twelve asphalt tiles with the glue on the back. And I turned them upside down and arranged them so it looked like a landscape. It's been in many art shows and it's called "Nebraska Landscape."

I had a piece of wood, took an axe, chopped it in many little pieces, burned it with a torch, polished it, waxed it, and then I reassembled it—it looked like a forest, it looked like people talking. I call it "Forest Conversation." It's in a museum in Kansas now.

My wife saved lint for quite a few years, and I made about 36 things out of lint. I had a show in Lincoln, Nebraska, of my lint things. Lint is beautiful stuff.

I had access to wonderful pieces of metal from a tail pipe factory in Seward that are twisted and curved. We did a piece of sculpture for a high school in Lincoln, Nebraska, a couple of years ago.

My wife and I refuse to give candy on Halloween at our house. One year the lumberyard had a box of little triangular pieces of wood. I took the wood and used rubber bands to put them together in bunches of six and seven. I painted some of the pieces and gave them out on Halloween. The parents couldn't deal with it, but their kids could. That week I got many telephone calls from parents telling me how their kids were so intrigued by those pieces of wood that they played all week with them.

One day I opened a cardboard box and found an empty jar of tempera paint from one of my former students. I asked, "Why is she sending me an empty jar of paint?" I looked inside and I saw the cracked paint had made a beautiful design. I thought, "Ah-ha, she looked inside of a jar and she thought of me, and she sent it to me." It pleases me that she thought of me when she looked in that jar, but what a risky thing it was for her to look into a jar when no one was looking.

In the picture of a windshield of a car, the man on the outside says, "The cracks in the glass are white." The man on the inside says, "You're wrong; they're black." If these two people don't change their point of view, they'll argue when in fact they're both right. And this is the same broken glass, so it could be maybe five or six things.

So we all have a point of view, and we all have to make shifts. That's why my first slide is so ugly, because those big feet are glued down to their arrogant one point of view. That's why it's so bad. They wouldn't move, and we all know people like that.

When students draw snow, some make footprints dark and some make them white. Some are looking against the sun, some are looking with the sun. I can't tell students how to draw snow; I can only teach them how to see snow. They draw what they see. And one day I noticed that footprints went up instead of down, on cement. I grew a little bit that day, when I could accept footprints going up.

When leaves are young and fresh and just starting out, they're flat and dull and boring. But when they're old and dying, they are beautiful. Maybe there's something we haven't learned yet about life.

We all have a viewpoint of life; when we see patterns of death and dying, we are reminded of bad things. This is the same pattern, but it's in a greenhouse, and it's Easter. So these are beginnings. Each one of us goes through life with a gravestone mentality or a greenhouse mentality that colors everything we do and say.

In my picture of an old man in a wheelchair in a retirement home, he moves his wheelchair, slowly. It would be nice if he could look down at his shadow on the orange rug, and realize that he is changing the universe. He needs to know that he can still do that.

The other day I looked up the word "ordinary" in the dictionary. One of the definitions I found: "Ordinary: a clergyman appointed in England to give spiritual assistance to condemned criminals, and to prepare them for the ordeal of the death penalty." When we have killed our spectacular world with boredom, and we are condemned to die, not to worry: Reverend Ordinary will be there to give his blessing.

2

The Marginal

Nancy Klenk Hill

In 1961 President John Kennedy climbed to the top of the newly erected Berlin wall and proclaimed, *"Ich bin ein Berliner."* I am a Berliner. I am one of you, he said. He had gone to the margin of the Western world and had asserted solidarity between the most powerful country in the world and an isolated enclave. The leader of the mainstream had reached out and identified with the marginal.

This incident reminds us that the marginal has both human and architectural connotations. Marginal people—that is, those whom society has ignored, or pushed to the economic edge, or isolated politically—tend to live in marginal places; places that mark off boundaries: at the outskirts, on the fringes, beside the tracks, the rivers, the other side of the wall.

It will perhaps seem incongruous to speak of the marginal at a gathering of mainstream society in a place like the Hyatt Regency. Our mainstream meeting places often have regal names: Regency, Brown Palace, the Helmsley Palace, the Hilton, a name once associated with great wealth, as Trump is now. Is it not odd that this country with its revolutionary history, its antimonarchical mythology, should imitate royalty in its hostelry and convention halls? What do these royal names and the accompanying decor tell us? Why do we imitate palaces instead of, say, the New England meeting hall, the midwestern grange, or even the formerly ubiquitous barn? Those places spoke to

15

an egalitarian consciousness, a sense that a community was comprised of people not separated, at least architecturally, into sharply defined economic groups.

These glass chandeliers, flocked walls, shining tiles, plush carpet, and gilt crests are supposed to make us feel that we've arrived—that we've cross a threshold into a glamorous world—glamorous precisely because it is not accessible to everyone.

Some of those who are not welcome here are those who live in the neighborhood, or, more accurately, on the neighborhood—on the heating grates and streets of the neighborhood. They congregate in places that tend, unlike our places, to religious terminology: the Salvation Army, Jesus Saves, Samaritan House, the St. Francis Center. Marginal places for marginal people; places that are so sparsely furnished they cannot be said to be decorated at all.

These places are not far from us—in a walking city like London we would say they were within walking distance. But few even know of their existence. Or rather, we all know of their existence—we just don't see it. We will ourselves not to see it, or, if we do notice any of it or of them (how easily those indefinite pronouns suit our purpose here), we do so only in the sense that white southerners noticed the dwellings of their slaves. The *mudsill factor*, it has been called, a factor that implies the slaves being outside the entrance, beyond the doorstep, across the mudsill, a factor that enhances one's own status. Their being outside the mudsill, on the margins, makes us feel mainstream—maybe even regal—until we really look at the palatial decor surrounding us. Seen up close, studied with a connoisseur's eye, the decor of American hostelry has more glitz than gold. There's something overdone and tasteless in most of these places, as if the decorator were deliberately exaggerating the imitation of grandeur to impress the gullible—that is, us. Between Christmas and New Year's Day, I attended the Modern Language Association convention in New Orleans and spent two and a half days interviewing candidates in my Hilton suite. A Hilton suite sounds so impressive, doesn't it? But why do you suppose they decorated it with wallpaper sporting two-foot wide orange roses? Imagine sitting for two and a half days in a room with two-foot orange roses on the wall! I do not exaggerate, but the Hilton did.

No, it isn't in the swank hotels that one expects to find good taste. The real locus of tasteful design these days is the doctor's office and the hospital. Sleek, ultra-modern, mauve and gray tones—the decor bespeaks the latest, the most up-to-date. These are our modern shrines. Our pseudo-palatial hotels are a throwback to a royal past that never was. Our hospitals are decidedly of the technological present—and of the sci-fi future. In a culture that seems to value the body over everything else, the preservers of the body and the halls they inhabit are designed to inspire awe and veneration.

Particularly is that the case where the technology is the highest. My daughter recently had a test called Magnetic Resonance Imaging (MRI). A whole suite of offices has been built in the basement of University Hospital to accommodate this gigantic machine and those who pay homage to it. A nurse-receptionist guards the access to this precious piece of wizardry. She, unlike the nurses in any other part of the hospital I have visited, had plenty of time to chat with us and to initiate us into the mysteries that lay before us. A special video, complete with soothing voiceover and euphemistic language, explained: "you may hear some tapping sounds." My daughter reported that the constant, rapidly knocking noises nearly drove her mad during the hour she was lying in the machine. The suite included separate dressing rooms and bathrooms—all of course in the de rigeur mauve and gray with nary a cabbage rose in sight. When the attendants took my daughter into the testing room I watched with a shudder through the glass window. A huge metal cylinder nearly filled the dimly lit room. It was like looking into a Pharaoh's tomb. And the treasure from our pocketbook exacted by the machine also has its Pharaonic dimension—fortunately absorbed by insurance.

The modern hospital is not all high-tech, however. Its low-tech wing tends to be the place for the marginal, like Kaiser's Emergency Room at St. Joseph's Hospital, where I sat several months ago holding my grandson who was running a 102 degree fever. For four hours we waited among the rest of the marginal in a room overheated, overcrowded, but woefully understaffed. I couldn't tell you how the room was decorated because I couldn't see any of the furniture. It was all draped with bodies—seated on the chairs, on the tables, standing at the counter, between the furniture.

What does this difference in design and expenditure tell us about our society? Do we like what it says? Do we agree with the implicit priorities?

I must admit that my sitting that night in the Kaiser emergency room was not my first experience of feeling marginal. And I dare say many of you have had the experience, too. For though we gather here as mainstreamers in the Regency, we academics, artists, and nurses are among the marginal in our society, largely because of our interest in and concern for humanity.

The mayor in Christopher Fry's play, "The Lady's Not for Burning," says, "Humanity. . . . No one is going to let it interfere with anything serious. I use it with great discretion, I assure you" (p. 43). There speaks the bureaucratic mind, that which sees humanity as somehow interfering with one's duties—to do what? To serve humanity somehow—preferably in the abstract.

We whose job it is to teach, to create, to heal are those who are viewed as somehow out of step with "the real work" of the serious world, that is, making money. We are viewed with some suspicion because we are not preoccupied with financial advancement.

Business and industry think of themselves as building America, developing the housing, erecting the factories, throwing up the fast-food franchises—and tearing them down as soon as the bottom line shows red instead of black. They think of themselves as the builders and of us as but the caretakers—a small step above the cleaning crews who come into those cavernous office buildings after the working day.

But they are mistaken. The real architects are us, the people who work with, care for, and teach people. Unless we do our job well, unless we build well, no set of structures in any city will long be a source of pride—or income. Our responsibility is only the mental and physical health of those who do the work in our society.

A businessman recently said to me, "Well, of course, you get a modest salary: you like what you do"—an interesting cause-effect relation. Only a few years ago another businessman remarked to me, "I'm glad I have a job good enough that my wife doesn't have to work." Few can say that today. Such remarks and attitudes tend to marginalize the listener—that is, me.

If I have sometimes felt marginal vocationally, I have also felt it avocationally. When I visited a young mother in the Sun Valley Housing Project just north of here, tucked in below the sports stadiums, I was overwhelmed by the cultural gap between us—something I later expressed in a poem called "What Makes Her Laugh?"

> The steady rattle of sit-coms
> Sometimes brings a grin
> In the small house muslined
> Against disturbing light
> And the bold invasive sight
> Of swaggering youth
> Just beyond her thin window
> In the development squeezed
> Between the highway and the tracks
> And called, without humor, Sun Valley.

Her daughter snuggling close, too close
Draws a solicitous smile
And a worried explanation:
"She don't like to go outside—
"Be away from me—
"She just do these puzzles, over and over,
"Sit here by me, watching TV."

We grimace kindly, beings from an alien world,
Seeking the words that will bridge the gap,
And she says, "What really made me laugh
"Was my boyfriend (he work in the cemetery)
"Telling about carrying a coffin
"From one grave to another
"And the lid popped open
"And the body rolled right out on the ground.
"I couldn't help laughing when he told me."
We laugh politely, and when we leave
She gives us a quick, sad smile.
"Be careful," she says.

Her admonition, "be careful," shifted the boundaries. Though I had
entered her marginal neighborhood between the valley highway and
the railroad tracks feeling all too mainstream, I left feeling marginal:
wary, cautious, conscious of my appalling—and possibly dangerous—
ignorance of the area.

An even more dramatic shift of mental boundaries occurred when
I volunteered at the St. Francis Center just a few blocks from here. I
spent a morning at the entry desk, welcoming and registering as guests
the homeless of all ages and descriptions: some few in the stereotypical
costume: smelly, dirty, unkempt—but most scrubbed and clean, though
bearing marks of frostbite and violence—and a few wearing button-
down shirts and nice pants, looking as if they had somehow stepped off
the wrong bus and inadvertently landed at 23rd instead of 17th Street.
When the mailman stopped by, I recognized his distinction from the
guests only by his uniform. With a repairman I narrowly missed inviting
him to sign in only by catching the initials on his blue pocket. By then I
was painfully aware that I could no longer distinguish the marginal by
appearances only, and that I myself—professional degrees and mort-
gage payments notwithstanding—or maybe because of those very distinctions—could easily become marginal.

Recently at the St. Francis Center a volunteer working at the welcoming desk recognized a former colleague come in the door. The experience was painful for both of them—the recently marginalized and the mainstreamer suddenly perceiving how easily his status could trickle away.

Having moved so far along the continuum between mainstream and marginal, I now proclaim, in the spirit of John Kennedy, I am a Willy Bosket. I acknowledge my resemblance to this self-proclaimed monster, the man considered the most violent inmate in New York State, the 26-year-old who admits to having committed more than 2,000 crimes between the ages of 9 and 15, the man now in solitary confinement for the next 20 years in a cell with a plexiglass door like a caged animal.

I a Willy Bosket? I, a respectable woman professor twice his age, who has never been in more trouble with the law than getting a speeding ticket? The comparison is ludicrous, isn't it? I'm not so sure.

A few years ago I went to Stapleton Airport to pick up my 81-year-old mother. It was one of those strange October days that begins mild and suddenly plummets—on this day a 40-degree temperature drop within a few hours. In southern Germany such weather changes are permissible evidence in court to explain erratic behavior. I parked in the ramp, met my mother at the gate, got her luggage, and instructed her to remain seated near the door while I brought the car around. When I pulled up in front of the door a policeman stopped me and said, "You can't leave the car unattended." I replied that I was alone (as was obvious) and had to park just a few seconds while I went in for my mother. "No," he said, "you have to park in the ramp." I explained that I already had done so. My exasperation level reached, I left the car and raced in for my mother. Thirty seconds later, emerging with her luggage, I saw the cop putting a ticket on my windshield. I blew. I got in the car, tore the ticket in half, and threw it at his feet. He calmly said, "I'll give you another ticket for littering." I picked up the torn ticket, looked at his feet, and for one wild moment seriously entertained the idea of stuffing the ticket in his shoe.

Now that moment of passionate, angry response might have cost me dearly. Yet I hovered, if ever so briefly, on the edge of a dangerously foolish, physical response. And I did so as a well brought-up woman, middle-class, gainfully employed—with all the behavioral inhibitions of my class and social status and gender.

What if I, like Willy Bosket, had been brought up poor in Harlem? Or not brought up at all. Or confined, as he has been, in reformatories and prisons almost continuously since age 9. Would I not feel rage? Would I not say with him, "I am at war with the system?" Would I not say, "I laugh at this system because there ain't a damn thing that it can do to me except to deal with the monster it has created," as reported in the New York Times?

Willy, like me, is smart. Willy, unlike me, has had no positive way to express his intelligence. Instead it has turned inwards, gnawing at him, eating at him, filling him with rage. It isn't difficult for me to understand something of how he feels. He is my brother, the son of my—and your mother—Eve.

There but for the grace of God, we say, there I could stand. We might rather turn it around and say, there by our neglect, our marginalization of our own brothers and sisters stands Willy Bosket. No wonder I can identify with him; I have helped to create him.

Willy Bosket describes himself as a monster created by our society. I think he may be right. Lots of kids grow up poor in places like Harlem and do not turn into monsters. But why should anyone? Why do we turn aside as if we couldn't think of anything to do? Why is our response as a society the construction of more prisons rather than the construction of decent homes and safe streets and better schools? Why do we employ more prison guards rather than more social workers? Willy Bosket is forcing the system to treat him as someone special now, requiring extraordinary, round-the-clock observation. What might have happened had such attention, together with love, been lavished on him as a child?

What might have happened had we attended to Harlem's drug problem 30 years ago? Had we recognized their problem as our problem then, drugs might not be in the hands of our suburban children now. Instead we marginalized the blacks, as we are marginalizing AIDS victims now.

But the results of such marginalization affect those of us in the mainstream. Our main streets in our main cities are now places to be avoided rather than places to celebrate our communal life. Our community hospitals can no longer bear the burden of our neglect. Our children perform at lower and lower educational levels compared to children around the world. More and more of the lower middle class are slipping into the realm of the marginal. During the past eight years such class shifts occurred at an alarming rate—clearly as a result of government policy. We are becoming our priorities.

Deplorable as this state of affairs may be, it is also the case that a different policy, instituted by an energized and alarmed people, could turn things around. But that can only happen if we declare ourselves one with the marginal.

Why should we do this? Can't we just arm ourselves with AKAs and hunker down in our fortified shelters we once called homes on our fenced-off streets we once called neighborhoods? Our emergency rooms are already viewing themselves as MASH units—we have become not only our priorities—we have become our TV shows, which emulated our foreign wars. No problem. We'll adapt to the new circumstances.

But it isn't only for public safety and a renewed sense of community that we might rethink the problem of marginalization. It isn't just because we ourselves could so easily, in this economic climate, slip into the ranks of the marginal. The fact is, although we live in a country celebrated, especially by us, as number one in the world of nations, our beginnings were decidedly marginal. We began, after all, 300 years ago as a rag-tag bunch of misfits from the old country whose primary virtue was a reckless willingness to take risks. We were street people without streets. We lived in shelters, in dugouts, in log cabins, in sod houses. We were the expendable of Europe, those whose absence caused little interruption of the regular routine and less remorse. We were the cast-offs— even the criminals—we who now convene in the Regency.

While I was growing up I was, like most Americans, oblivious of all generations but my own. My mother's family took a keen interest in genealogy and had traced its origins back to the knights of King Arthur's Round Table. When I got to college I learned that my glorious English genealogy led back to nothing but myth. After college my husband and I went to Germany and I thought perhaps the German side of my genealogy would lead to something more substantial than the literary mists of Avalon. I was not disappointed, at least in a material sense. My German name, Klenk, turned out to mean doorhandle, which may explain my interest in the marginal and boundaries and doorsills. I come by it genealogically. Even worse was the discovery some years later that the earliest Klenk who could be traced had been not a musician, not a writer, not even a shadowy knight, but a day laborer.

The discovery makes me less comfortable with the Rockefellers and the Rothschilds, who seldom invite me for tea anyway, but it makes me a whole lot more comfortable with the Willy Boskets. My marginal great-great-grandfather made it possible for his sons and grandsons—and great-great-granddaughter—to become mainstream.

The pattern is a repeated one not only in our culture, but throughout history. That infusion of talent, of ambition, of drive keeps surging up from the marginal, renewing and refreshing and sometimes reordering, even replacing the mainstream. Think of the history of the Israelites, a marginal people if ever there were one—a tiny band of nomads wandering across the inhospitable reaches of the mid-east, guided by a god unseen and held in contempt by all the other nations of the region. But try to imagine the history of the world without Israel. Our Hebrew heritage is immense, and the outpouring of books, music, art, theorems, formulae, incalculable. Or consider the black culture in our own country. That marginalized people gave us the spiritual, blues, jazz—what we think of as an indigenous American sound—and they gave us a model of endurance justly celebrated in much of what ranks as best in American literature.

We need to realize that those marginal groups, those people at the fringes of the social fabric, holding on to the remnants of civilized life by a fraying thread, are the very people who can call us to account and make us realize who we are. It is the marginal, not the mainstream, that finally defines the nature of a society.

Literature has long acknowledged this fact. It is, indeed, the element that makes literature often so subversive, or at least seemingly subversive to whatever establishment is currently in power. The phenomenon can be seen in literature's treatment of "the other" in whatever context it may appear: women in a male-dominated society, blacks in a white-dominated society, the people of God in a heathen society.

Literature deals preeminently with the marginal. Homer's *Odyssey* and *Iliad* established a mythology that enabled a small assemblage of Hellenic city-states to exert as much power over the imagination as did that other marginal people, the Hebrews, at the end of the Mediterranean. Jesus was rejected as marginal by most of the Jews, yet came to be recognized as fulfilling the Biblical text: "the stone that the builders rejected has become the cornerstone." Dante wrote the Divine Comedy in exile from his beloved Florence. Dickens repeatedly returned to the mean streets of his marginal childhood in novels that have remained best sellers for 150 years. In the novel he called his "favorite child," David Copperfield remembers his own experience as the marginal in order to quicken his own and his readers' sense of compassion. Toni Morrison in *Beloved* does something similar through a process she calls rememory, bringing to consciousness those suppressed incidents of slavery, not to relive the suffering or to reignite indignation against the enslavers, but to redeem both the sufferers and those who caused them to suffer. *Beloved* is a healing book, one which makes clearer than any other book I can think of, what is positive about being marginal, and why the marginal must be acknowledged and embraced. It is, simply, to make us whole. In a world where some were masters, some slaves, where some are healthy, some ill—even with AIDS or cancer, where some are young and some will be old, we must acknowledge ourselves in all. Otherwise, we marginalize ourselves. We say, in effect, we are masters, healthy, young—and we look with disdain on those who do not share our self-proclaimed virtues. We also look with fear, for we know our present power, health, and youth will not last.

There is a simple way to stave off that fear of becoming marginal that allows us to make others marginal. It is to embrace them as ourselves.

Of all the professions, none is better situated to do this than are nurses. Your assistance, your healing, your gracious acceptance of the marginal as human beings brings them back into the human community—and restores a sense of community for us all.

For we are all, finally, marginal. We are but sojourners on this planet earth, and we are making our way home—though most of us have forgotten where that is. To quote again from *The Lady's Not for Burning,* Margaret says, "Have any of you seen that poor child Alizon? I think she must be lost." Nicholas replies, "Who isn't? The best thing we can do is to make wherever we're lost in look as much like home as we can" (p. 82). It's a good suggestion for making do with the interim situation in which we live. But it also suggests that home is something other than the place we return to each night.

At the end of this wonderful play Thomas says to Jennet, "I have to see you home, though neither of us knows where on earth it is." The lines imply that home is not to be found on earth—only the search for it. And that idea has vast implications for the way we live our lives and help others to live, as well as to end, theirs.

Two recent news stories bear odd connection to our topic. In Chicago, Rodolfo Linares held hospital staff at gunpoint while he unplugged the life-support equipment attached to his 15-month-old son, then cradled the baby until he died. The baby had been plugged in, and brain-damaged, since August. "I'm not here to hurt anyone. I'll only hurt you if you try to plug my baby back in," he said.

In Boulder a Benedictine nun, a founder of St. Walburga's Abbey, died peacefully in her sleep at age 89. Sister Simone said, "It is not a sad occasion for us. When you work all your life to be close to God, death is not sad. We call it going home."

Going home. Not sad. How many people outside the two abbeys in the country can say that about death? Why are we as a society so hooked on life-preservation machinery? We seem to expect doctors to delay the process of our heading home, to maintain us in the mainstream as long as possible, to make us forget our essential marginality. We have thereby made priests of our doctors and shrines of our hospitals, pretending in our modern myth of longevity that if the body can just be maintained, everything will be all right.

Until quite recently a standard response of the young to the question, "How ya doin?" was "maintainin'." We, with the assistance of the medical profession, are maintainin'. And that myth feeds ever greater expenditures for technological means to extend our bodily life. A guest at the St. Francis Center recently put a different twist on the standard question, "How ya doin?" "Without," he said.

No two words express more succinctly what I have been trying to say about the marginal and our relation to them. Are we to continue "maintainin'" while others do "without"? Are we to continue expending vast treasure on the maintenance of our mortal bodies while others have no health care at all? Do we as a culture really believe that some of our bodies are worth preserving at any cost, while other bodies are worth no cost at all? What is next? Freezing the body for unthawing at a later stage of medical history? Embalming and preservation in glass tombs like that of Lenin? Why are we so enamoured of the body and so afraid of death? Is it because we really have forgotten the way home? "Show me the way to go home. I'm tired and I want to go home," the song says.

Acknowledging our mutual marginality would, I believe, restore our perspective and help us to reorder our priorities. I offer a five-point twist on a familiar syllogism as my parting shot, not because it is logical (for it is not), but because these points are linked to each other irrevocably.

1. We are all marginal, that is, mortal.

2. Being marginal/mortal we will eventually die, medicine or no medicine, hospital or no hospital.

3. We will then return home, from whence we came. As Wordsworth puts it in his ode, "Intimations on Immortality," "Trailing clouds of glory do we come from God, who is our home."

4. While we are experiencing this brief, marginal, earthly episode, it is incumbent on us to care about and for each other.

5. Sometimes doctors, and occasionally technology, but mostly nurses care for us. They are therefore not at the margin, but at the center of human caring.

I think it could be argued that nurses are what holds this society together—sometimes, as when they assist at an operation, quite literally so. Their minute-by-minute attention to us when we have become ill, and therefore marginal, enables us to return to the mainstream. Though the doctors function as the high priesthood and collect the princely salaries, the nurses are usually the ones who win our affection for being there when we need them. They are the ones who humanize medicine for us, who make us feel we are something more than another body to be processed and stamped. They are the ones who have time for us, and who patiently explain and translate what the doctor has hastily said or, worse, written. They are the ones who hold our hands, engage our eyes, calm our hearts when we confront some new process or some new machine.

But it cannot be easy dealing with the marginal each working day and being treated as marginal oneself by the doctors. Furthermore, the margins of the marginal seem to be extending. While all the ill are in some ways marginal, the very sick and those with socially unacceptable diseases are even more so. And to nurse the most marginal, those about to die, must be difficult indeed. For one cannot do that without facing, daily, one's own mortality.

This all takes a lot of what, growing up in the midwest, we called character. It was a quality thought to be particularly developed by such things as having to go to the outhouse in the middle of a winter night— or of somehow managing not to go. Such character builds steel—a tough, no-nonsense approach to this world, and I have known nurses for whom sickness is a moral failing—a failure of character. Families of such nurses do not get sick. They do not dare.

This facing the marginal and our shared marginality finally requires humor—the capacity to recognize in our precarious human condition the presence of the comic sense. In my favorite play by Fry (p. 52) from which I have quoted so frequently, Thomas says to Jennet,

> Are you going to be so serious
> About such a mean allowance of breath as life is?
> We'll suppose ourselves to be caddis-flies
> Who live one day. Do we waste the evening
> Commiserating with each other about
> The unhygienic condition of our worm-cases?
> For God's sake, shall we laugh?

Jennet responds, For what reason?

> For the reason of laughter; since laughter is surely
> The surest touch of genius in creation.
> Would you ever have thought of it, I ask you,
> If you had been making man, stuffing him full

Of such hopping greeds and passions that he has
To blow himself to pieces as often as he
Conveniently can manage it—would it also
Have occurred to you to make him burst himself
With such a phenomenon as cachinnation?
That same laughter, madam, is an irrelevancy
Which almost amounts to revelation.

We are but caddis-flies, here but briefly, recognizing ourselves as marginal, and we can either spend our brief time commiserating with each other about our marginality, what Fry calls "the unhygienic condition of our worm-cases" or we can burst ourselves with cachinnation, with laughter.

For God's sake, shall we laugh?

REFERENCES

Fry, C. (1977). *The lady's not for burning.* New York: Oxford.

Monster is caged for life and jailers stand back. (April 17, 1989). *New York Times*, p. 1.

3

The Tensions and Passions of Caring

Maxine Greene

I want to begin with an affirmation, indeed a celebration, of the recognition of caring as the ground of ethical existence. I believe deeply that reflective practice in the human services ought to begin in a consciousness of situatedness, particularity, feeling, and concern. Therefore, I cannot but hope that more and more practitioners will respond to the "caring imperative" and think what it means to choose themselves in accord with its demands.

All of us are aware, nevertheless, that caring refers to a spectrum of human experiences, emotions, and ways of being in the world. I am going to talk about some of the tensions in efforts we ourselves make to be caring and to provoke other human beings to care. These are efforts not unlike the ones we exert to move persons to thoughtfulness, to attentiveness to the world, and perhaps to the desire to transform it. We know well the extremes to which people will go to take refuge on occasion in stock responses, passivity, in what Milan Kundera calls "kitsch" or the erection of "folding screens" to curtain off reality (1984, pp. 248–249) even as so many take refuge in indifference, distancing, unconcern.

The tensions are intensified by the fact that we are talking about care in a fearfully careless society. Administered, systematized, bureaucratized, violent as it is, such a society requires of us a deliberate resistance to many of its dominant values. I have in mind, particularly, the prevalent privatism and self-involvement, as I do certain kinds of cold manipulative expertise. At once, we are challenged to learn to look toward an unpredictable future, to experience the peculiar passion that opens toward untapped possibility.

Martin Buber used to write about the degree to which modern people submerge themselves in collectivities, and how important it has become to rescue themselves from a collectivism "which devours all selfhood" (1957, pp. 110–111). He did not, obviously, have what we conceive of as community in mind or what we think of as human connectedness. He meant a "bundling together," where there is an "organized atrophy of personal existence" rather than a "confirmation in life lived towards one another" (p. 31). But he believed that, when that occurs, persons are likely to feel pain in the distortion of the relation to themselves, pain they keep trying to dull. Doing this, they suppress desire as well.

Buber said that the genuine educator's first task was "to keep the pain awake, to waken the desire" (p. 111). This is part of what I have in mind when I speak of the "passions" of caring, paradoxical though it may seem. I have wide-awakeness in mind; I have in mind a going up against the abstract, the domesticating, the systematized. Only then are there likely to be the collaborative actions intended to transform. I believe that caring must be deliberately achieved, as freedom must be achieved. It is going to take thoughtfulness, courage, and desire to do so—an opening of spaces where we can truly care. It is going to take political action now and then within and outside our institutions. And it may take poetry and serendipitous visions, and music, and even painting for the sake of empowering persons to hear and see what is often behind the veil.

Caring undoubtedly involves the capacity to grasp the lived reality of other living persons, to help those others grow in their own authentic fashions, or to attain a well-being of which they may be deprived. It involves the capacity, as Nel Noddings says, to regard another's reality as possible for oneself. Viewing another that way, we experience the need for action "to eliminate the intolerable . . . to fill the need, to actualize the dream" (1984, p. 14). We cannot objectify those others about whom we presume to care. We cannot look at them as if they were merely "cases," or as if their existential realities were defined by role, diagnosed illness, income, or test score. This means, for many of us, a feeling of strain, of uneasiness. We have to resist the temptation (sometimes the benevolent temptation) to classify, categorize, label once and for all; since we realize that we must resist it if we wish to enter some dialogical relation with others, if we are to feel others' possibilities as our own.

In Melville's "Bartleby the Scrivener," the lawyer-narrator desperately desires to categorize the stranger who refuses to act in accord with "convention and usage." Bartleby keeps saying, "I prefer not to," driving his employer nearly to madness because he does not dare to share the scrivener's forlorn world. Finding Bartleby in his Wall Street office of a Sunday, the narrator writes: "Before, I had never experienced aught but a not unpleasing sadness. The bond of a common humanity now drew me irresistibly to gloom. A fraternal melancholy! For both I and Bartleby were sons of Adam" (1986, p. 111). He recalls the happy crowds on Broadway, ponders Bartleby's aloneness, has a presentiment of the scrivener's "Pale form . . . laid out, among uncaring strangers in its shivering winding sheet." He tries vainly to make Bartleby leave and finally moves his business to another office in his frustration. He is eventually summoned back by the new tenants to do something about the clerk who will not leave. He allows him to be arrested as a vagrant and taken to the Tombs; and, when Bartleby prefers not to eat and dies, the lawyer concludes his tale with a futile utterance of something resembling care: "Ah, Bartleby!", he says, "Ah, humanity!" (p. 130). Yes, it is an account of marginality and of fearful separation, of groping on two sides for care. Melville knew profoundly how many solitary "bachelors" there were in a country devoted to laissez-faire and exchange values, a nation of calculations and formulations and barren walls. He knew how little coming together there was in Wall Street offices and paper factories and on whaling ships; and he still makes us strain (as he must have strained) against the limits set up by our shared realities.

We have, of course, learned from women writers like Nancy Chodorow, Carol Gilligan, and many others that women are less frequently walled away in free enterprise zones than men, less prone to the isolate's or the manager's kind of forlornness. This is because we have been more likely to live lives as contextualized beings, in networks of relationships, whether chosen or not. If there are multiple threads that connect us to those around us, we cannot easily take the vantage point of the outside observer, the inspector, the formulator. We have learned that, in part because of such connectedness, women's moral judgments tend to be linked to feelings of empathy and compassion, rather than to formal rational principles transcending the multifaceted, contingent, intersubjective world in which we are embedded or engaged. Gilligan views the ideal of care itself as "an activity of relationship, of seeing and responding to need, taking care of the world by sustaining the web of connection so that no one is left alone" (1981, p. 62).

This association between gender qualities and morality is probably related to the discrepancies in the kinds of worlds in which men and women have been expected to operate. The male world of work in the corporate and governmental domains has long required, it is now recognized, an adherence to methods and procedures that abstract from personal attachment, inclination, and concern for *particular* other people. If we take a historical point of view, we recognize that personal attachment and concern were appropriate to what were thought of as women's distinctive spheres, as those spheres were defined since the Industrial Revolution. That revolution, coupled with the emergence of the nation-state, led to reliance on nonpersonal law as the primary ordering principle in the economic and public domains. It was then that compliance with the nonpersonal and the abstract, with contractual relations and the rest, began to be clearly associated with masculine traits.

Men, after all, were the ones who moved into the clattering spaces of the factories, into offices and shops, into legislative and assembly halls. They were the ones who officially exerted power, who administered (classified, controlled, and protected) the inhabitants of whatever they considered to be *their* world. If they were decent people, they tried to live by principle—to be fair, to be impartial with regard to groups or aggregates of nameless people whose faces they seldom saw. Even in factories like the Lowell mills, where the work force was largely female, male operatives dominated and excluded women workers, going so far as to refuse them entry into the early trade unions.

The part played by teachers (who, after all, were mainly women) in the structured and formulated spheres of public schools became exemplary, even for nursing education. The school systems were invented and developed primarily by male reformers and administrators. They took the place of "dame schools" and other small voluntary schools where the values and intimacies of home life pervaded the atmosphere. Inequalities, it is true, were rampant. Thousands of children did not go to school at all. The teachers were not professional in any modern sense; and there was no assurance that the kind of literacy required to bind persons into community would be effectively conveyed. In the name of the "common," nevertheless, and the "public," the systems were conceptualized in nonpersonal, apparently equitable terms. The language used to argue for them was a language geared to generalized concerns: social control, adjustment, Americanization, measurable achievement, basic skills. After all, they deal with youth *in general*—strangers who had to be socialized if a reliable social order were to be created and maintained.

In spite of this, teachers (like nursing educators later on) were and are engaged in situation-specific undertakings involving diverse and specific human beings, not people in general, persons variously responsive to the demands of adjustment and control (Schon, 1983, p. 329). Encountering such beings in face-to-face relationships, many teachers could not but try to provoke dialogues, to understand thinking processes, to help students understand their own confusions, to stimulate questioning. In other words, they could not but try to care. Granted, they did so with differing degrees of warmth and attentiveness. Today, many still feel bound to teach to tests; others teach in accord with disciplinary norms; still others try to move learners to take initiatives and teach themselves. There is a spreading recognition that, whatever the atmosphere or the themes of instruction, the focus ought not always to be on children in the aggregate, or on the "third grade," or on the "hyperactive" as a category, or on the "gifted," or the "slow." More attention ought to be paid to living persons in their particularity.

Professionals continue trying to chart the situations in which they work, to find guiding principles that govern them, so that they will not be continually figuring out what they have to do. But it is only in changing, uncharted situations that caring acts can be initiated in an authentic sense. Only in such situations, many will admit, do persons *qua* persons live in a "we-relation" to one another, "make music together," as one philosopher put it, using the metaphor of a string quartet (Schutz, 1964, p. 159). It is in such circumstances that attention is paid to the specific tonality, to the blink of an eye, to the permutations of emerging sound. Listening, looking from the ground of shared artistry, those involved know full well that they are in a domain of possibility. Firm predictions about what they produce can never be made. They can only begin over and over, pay heed, open themselves to one another. In an atmosphere of intensity and care, music no one could precisely anticipate will come to be.

Musicians, of course, do not have to suffer the demands of a system quite as directly as do nurses and teachers. Much like nurses, who have to be acquainted with the requirements of triage, the demands of diagnosis related groups (DRGs), or the rules governing an emergency room, even the most caring teachers have to react to the demands issuing from the bureaucracy: testing procedures, attendance regulations, scheduling, and the rest. If they cannot somehow decipher what Hannah Arendt described as a mode of dominion best characterized as "rule by Nobody" (1972, p. 137), the bureaucracy in which they work is often likely to affect practitioners as a great silencing weight of

prescriptions and prohibitions. Because they frequently cannot identify who precisely is responsible, they feel themselves subordinated to a
given, something as natural and unarguable as the law of gravity.
There is something incapacitating about the pressure, as there is something overwhelming about the technical rationality that presumably
makes it work.

On one level, most professionals realize that technical rationality and
the research generalizations to which it gives rise offer sources of insight, reservoirs of knowledge. No one can toss aside what is being
found out with regard to the AIDS virus, chemotherapy, or radiation.
At once, no one can simply assume that the results of such discovery or
the methodology of the research can be applied in the particular encounters of hospital life. It is the same with classroom teachers: generalizations about cognition, mastery, thinking repertoires, and the like
cannot be put to use in classrooms without shared reflection, improvisa-
tory work, open-ended efforts to provoke diverse people to find their
own voices and make their own kind of sense. In both cases, a reflective
and creative consciousness must be at work as awareness grows of obstacles, determinates, and systematic constraints. And, indeed, there must
be such an awareness, linked with the imaginative capacity to posit
alternatives. If we are to respond to the imperative of care, we need to
ponder what it signifies to open more benign spaces in our institutions,
especially those governed by the latest ethos of technology. There ought
to be spaces where people can make music together and where many
different kinds of choices can be made and different languages discovered. It is in those spaces, I am convinced, that care must be pursued.

Pondering the meeting places of technique and care, I recall a recent
novel, Christa Wolf's *Accident: A Day's News* (1989). It takes place on the
day in which the disaster at Chernobyl becomes known in Germany; it is
also the day when the beloved brother of the narrator is having a deli-
cate brain operation. We are presented, therefore, with technology in
its two aspects: destruction released by carelessness; restorative action
at the service of care. The book deals with fusion rather than fission,
with an effort to create some order in a disrupted experience. Near the
beginning, the narrator is talking to her daughter, asking her to tell her
about the children. She writes about the terrible pictures surging up in
her mind.

> I was once more forced to admire the way in which everything fits
> together with a sleepwalker's precision: the desire of most people
> for a comfortable life, their tendency to believe the speakers on

raised platforms and the men in white coats; the addiction to harmony and the fear of contradiction of the many seem to correspond to the arrogance and hunger for power, the dedication to profit, unscrupulous inquisitiveness and self-infatuation of the few. So what was it that didn't add up in this equation? (p. 17).

She turns to the children, to the look of grass, to the concreteness and beauty of the earth, the sky. At the end, when she hears that her brother has survived, she says, "How difficult it would be, brother, to take leave of this earth." The book not only reveals an outcry audible behind the prose, but also the ways in which connections are identified: pollution, milk, green grass, little children, nuclear energy, microsurgery, the art of writing, sisterly care, a cherishing of the earth.

Yes, of course, it is a woman speaking; and, indeed, it is a woman's way of knowing. But I do not want to suggest that technologists or systems or scientific inquiries are, by their very nature, inexorably male, nor that a predominantly female world would eliminate them or ensure their beneficence. Because classrooms, like hospital rooms and clinics, have to such a large extent been women's spheres, there are sometimes suggestions that, if they were extended somehow, if the mutuality and relatedness that mark them were to become potent enough to replace competitiveness and impersonal planning, natural gardens of care and concern would bloom. We not only have to cope with the tension of living in bureaucratized circumstances, governed by values like effectiveness and efficiency, we must deliberately challenge the compliance with "men in white coats" on the part of women as well as men. Even as we strive for the personal encounter, the meeting of eyes, the caring *for,* we have to struggle for the true word behind the artificial talk. We have to exert ourselves to construct corridor communities and, eventually, public spaces. Care, more and more of us are coming to know, cannot be conceived of mainly as a way of relating to those in the intimate circles of our lives. It can become a feeling, impassioned mode of thrusting into a resistant world together, a mode of remaking lived situations and devising meaningful projects in the face of obstacles that have to be named and surmounted if caring is to be achieved.

Even though I grant their significance as touchstones and reference points, experiences of caring and being cared for do not strike me as being necessarily universal. Nor are they given in every human career. Nor is caring, except in its natural expression, to be expected of everyone. It is not a way of being (or feeling, or acting) that simply happens if we, especially those of us who are women, are left to ourselves. I think of the unhappy lives I know: those of the single mothers, the desperate adolescent mothers who abandon their children in hospitals; those of the addicted, old and young; those of homeless women, once the sustainers of their families, on the streets. The caring imperative has to be integrated with an imperative to reweave the torn networks of relationship in neighborhoods, to restructure the support systems destroyed by carelessness and greed.

As we confront what our recent political history has signified, we might also confront the differences between those who take an essentialist view with regard to women (that is, the view that makes certain values and virtues distinctive of a female "essence") and those who treat gender as a function of certain social and cultural situations susceptible to eventual change. It is true enough that under certain conditions of oppression, women have developed—more than they might have otherwise—strengths and attributes many people admire and want to promote, especially in the fragmented, privatized, hyperorganized world of today. We do not have to be reminded how mothering and family responsibilities continue to encourage capacities for caring in interpersonal ways, as they have made clear the connection between such ways of being and feeling for those who are near and dear. Most of us recognize that without warmth of feeling to start with, we would not exert ourselves for the sake of others as much as we do.

It is easy to see, in fact, why—in the midst of everyday life which resembles a desert or a wasteland or a running track for many people— loneliness and compulsiveness have given rise to a spectrum of notions of the way things in a nurturing world ought to be. Some of these ideas come from memories or fantasies; others arise in counterformation to present experiences of abandonment or solitude.

Linda Alcoff has reminded us that, determined as we are to create a more caring, decent, and humane society, we must be wary of promoting the conditions that gave rise to the valued attributes and modes of conduct in the first place—"forced parenting, lack of physical autonomy, dependence for survival on mediation skills" (1988, p. 267). Anyone of us might extend the list to include conditions prevalent in nursing and in teaching. Like Alcoff, however, we ought to ask "What conditions for women do we want to promote? A freedom of movement such that we can compete in the capitalist world alongside men? A continued restriction to child-centered activities? To the extent cultural feminism merely valorizes genuinely positive attributes developed under oppression, it cannot map our future long-range course." I would want to stress this, especially in connection with "the caring imperative."

To put too exclusive an emphasis on the virtues developed under oppression would be like celebrating what Friedrich Nietzsche called "slave values" that inverted the artistocratic value equations "good/noble/powerful/beautiful/happy/favored-of-the-gods" (1956, p. 167). That inversion meant that "only the poor, the powerless, are good; only the suffering, sick, and ugly, truly blessed. His concern was that oppressed, underprivileged, impotent people, to stay safe and in the good graces of those who dominated them, kept affirming and trying to live by values like humility and uncomplaining acceptance. I do not want caring to imply these things; I want it to be vital, assertive, immodest, and sometimes (for good reason) indignant.

This reminds me of Alice Walker's Miss Celie in *The Color Purple* writing her letters to God: "I am fourteen years old. I have always been a good girl. Maybe you can give me a sign letting me know what is happening to me" (1982, p. 11). I know people have mixed feelings about Nietzsche; but his point remains important for the crushed Celies of the world and for those who are nurses and teachers, committed to care. Walker's character is fortunate enough to meet a blues singer named Shug Avery, who serves as her Nietzsche. You may remember Celie, after a long time, trying to chase "that old white man out of my head." She says,

> I been so busy thinking bout him I never truly notice nothing God make. Not a blade of corn (How it do that?) not the color purple (where it come from?) Not the little wildflowers. Nothing. Now that my eyes are opening, I feels like a fool. Next to any little scrub of a bush in my yard, Mr. _____'s evil sort of shrink. But not altogether. Still, it is like Shug say, You have to git man off your eyeball, before you can see anything a'tall. Man corrupt everything, say Shug. He on your box of grits, in your head, and all over the radio. He try to make you think he everywhere. Soon as you think he everywhere, you think he God. But he ain't. Whenever you trying to pray, and man plop himself on the other end of it, tell him to git lost, say Shug. Conjure up flowers, wind, water, a big rock. But this hard work, let me tell you. He been there so long, he don't want to budge. He threaten lightning, floods and earthquakes. Us fight. I hardly pray at all. Every time I conjure up a rock, I throw it. Amen" (pp. 178–179).

She has to reflect, imagine, resist. She has to deal with the oppressive power she calls "man." I would affirm that it was only when her eyes begin to open that she can care, authentically and with dignity.

This is not, of course, to say that humility and modesty are intrinsically bad and to be rejected. It does mean that we ought not to select

those characteristics, even those virtues, that were particularly responsive to our felt plight as women professionals and treat them as guides or
norms along the way. Alcoff, warning against essentialism, says we are
always in danger of "solidifying an important bulwark of sexual oppression: the belief in an 'innate womanhood' to which we must all adhere lest
we be deemed either inferior or not 'true' women" (1988, p. 266).

The other side must not be neglected. It is the case that an often
joyous sense of self-discovery and self-affirmation has accompanied the
recognition that "women's ways of knowing" (Belenkey et al., 1987), so
long derided as soft, childish, and not truly cognitive, are important and
have to be granted their own integrity. Many have taken pride in the
delayed acknowledgment of relational thinking, in the breaking through
of disciplinary boundaries, in a "blurring of the genres" that is in large
measure due to women's scholarship. The new visibility of women's perspectives and the ongoing opening of those perspectives have exposed
the partiality and deficiencies of countless modes of sense-making—in
history, science, literary criticism, the various forms of art. What woman
cannot applaud the disclosures Barbara McClintock has made us comprehend, or the insights Evelyn Fox Keller has provoked in her *Gender
and Science* inquiry? I think not only of Nel Noddings but also of Jean
Baker White, Carol Gilligan, Nancy Chodorow, Barbara Ehrenreich,
Sara Ruddick, and so many others. I think of what Sandra Gilbert and
Susan Gubar helped me see in *The Madwoman in the Attic,* of how Linda
Nochlin has opened up paintings and sculptures, of what Catharine
Stimpson has shown us about the Golden Age of Greece and the Renais-
sance, not to speak of the canons governing the humanities.

I particularly relish what Martha Nussbaum has done in *The Fragility
of Goodness* (1986) when, in her rereading of Greek classic texts, she
opposes flexibility and responsiveness to rigidity, and when she affirms
so clearly the fundamental value of community and friendship in ethical
experience (p. 70). But these are instances of peculiar power and illumi-
nations hidden for too many generations, often forced underground.
Now that they are being released and brought into play by (mainly)
women thinkers, they are generating all sorts of new and wider visions.
This, however, can happen only if they work to amplify, to renew,
rather than bringing new dualisms into being.

Many of us have learned that it is not enough to concentrate on
offsetting the misogyny, the blindness, the carelessness in our culture
and in the institutions where we work. Nor is it enough to single out
only those perspectives that have been repressed and give them superior status in the intellectual and political spheres. We must keep asking

ourselves about the degree to which we ignore distinctions and diversities, whether we sometimes shut off existential possibilities, even for ourselves. What do we do, when we think about caring, with regard to Henry James's Isabel Archer, the women managers we meet, all of those who do not fit our relational and caring ideal?

Our need for our own identity, writes Elizabeth Young-Bruehl, is primarily a need not to be dictated to or dominated. But that ought not to suppress what she calls "our internal conversations, and especially the unwelcome conflicts in them and the archaic voices in them" (1988, p. 21). She wants to see us thinking in many modalities. She challenges us to listen to all the voices in our minds for the sake of achieving not *an* identity "but a more communicative form of life—the possibility of conversational reconciling, both in ourselves and others." She says, finally, that we internalize and must internalize exemplary men and women, that we need ego ideals of both sexes, "but it is women who were marginalized and continued thinking with whom we associate our own marginalized desires to know" (p. 22).

The imperative to care, especially for teachers, recalls the multiple conversations that must be heeded in our classrooms, the "heteroglossia" that characterizes them, and the ways in which they make us aware of the sounds of so many voices within ourselves. Indeed, I am eager to enter into the kinds of dialogues with young people that might overcome marginality and create some sort of reciprocity. We hope to avoid the monologism of power; we want, as we try to act on the caring we experience, to reveal not only the course of our own critical thinking and judgment. We want to make visible somehow our incompleteness, our own internal dialogues.

Teaching, in one dimension, is the kind of action intended to provoke newcomers or younger persons to pose their own questions, to go in search. Caring for those persons in the course of teaching is, in a certain respect, to lend them some of our lives. What we do is try to make accessible and learnable not merely the knacks, the rudiments, the tricks of the trade. We try to disclose the many ways there are of interpreting the experienced world. We try to create situations that will allow for the expression of a range of intelligences, and we try to provide opportunities for the release of imagination so that learners can strive for what lies beyond, what represents some meaningful possibility. In a classroom, a teacher cannot care intimately or on a level of mutuality for every person. Even so, one teacher can do more than care *about* various individuals outside the ring of immediate concern.

A consideration of principles, like those of fairness or impartiality or

ordinary decency, seems appropriate. An attentiveness to such generalized prescriptions, along with some felt obligation to live according to
them, need not dilute the kinds of moral action based on care. In fact,
obligation may be what opens the path to caring. The play *Professional
Foul*, by Tom Stoppard, deals with a philosophy convention taking place
in Prague at the same time as a soccer match. Professor Anderson, a
British analytic philosopher, is accosted by a former student, Hollar,
who asks him to smuggle a thesis on human rights to England when the
convention is over. On principle, the professor refuses at first, saying
there is an etiquette about visiting a foreign country, a norm he cannot
defy. He discovers later that Hollar's house has been searched after
their encounter, that the young man has been arrested; and Anderson, a
professor of ethics, is forced to confront the man's wife and child.
Beginning to consider the principle of regard for human rights, he
unexpectedly revises the speech he had planned to make and had
passed through the censors. He speaks now about how ethics was long
considered a kind of monument constructed of platonic entities like
honesty, loyalty, fairness, all of which provided norms against which we
could measure our behavior. In recent times, he tells his audience, the
idea of justice has been thought to have no meaning outside of linguistic
usage; it consists only of the ways in which we use the word. Then:

> And common observation shows us that this view demands qualifica-
> tion. A small child who cries "that's not fair" when punished for
> something done by his brother or sister is apparently appealing to an
> idea of justice which is, for want of a better word, natural. And we
> must see that natural justice, however illusory, does inspire many
> people's behavior much of the time. As an ethical utterance it seems
> to be an attempt to define a sense of rightness which is not simply
> derived from some other utterance elsewhere (1978, pp. 117–118).

There is, the philosopher says, a "sense of right and wrong that precedes utterance . . . individually experienced." And then he makes
the point that that sense of right and wrong concerns one person's
dealing with another. Taking the path of intuition, he comes to a
conclusion that connects the sense of right and wrong to caring, in the
way we have been using the term. Whether or no, Professor Anderson
could only act on his feeling of concern for his student and his student's little boy when he could appeal to—or *find*—a principle of
fairness. This in no way lessened the moral quality of his choice, it
seems to me; nor did it reduce his feelings of concern, mixed as they

were with compassion and responsibility and care. In the end, he does find a way of secreting Hollar's document out of Prague—an act he now believes to be wholly right.

We teachers are most likely to act out our feelings of care if we have extended our concerns for equality, justice, and liberty to include more persons than those in our immediate vicinity. When this happens, we may be more capable of opening spaces where all sorts of learners can make their voices audible and their faces visible, where they can be heard and seen striving to enter the conversation—coming together to shape visions of the way things ought to be. What such diverse people disclose as they plan for the future may thwart or even defy what their teachers desire or approve. Caring for the young in an open society means introducing them to shared conceptions of what is right and what is good, even as it means releasing them to do unpredictable things. Of course it also means providing as many resources as possible, offering entry points to the multiple fields of study. Like Hannah Arendt, I believe that education

> is where we decide whether we love our children enough not to expel them from our world and leave them to their own devices, nor to strike from their hands their chance of undertaking something new, something unforeseen by us, but to prepare them in advance for the task of renewing a common world (1961, p. 196).

With that in mind, I still remain deeply interested in the concreteness of things and the particularities of that common world. In the spaces I hope we can open, I would want to see persons becoming vividly present to one another in the encounters and in their quests. Part of the caring imperative is to struggle against the temptation to distance, to make objects out of students or patients or clients. Martin Heidegger thought that care refers to a structure of concern characterizing all human consciousness, one of the ways there are of grasping what presents itself in the faces of others and of the world. Crucially, however, it entails a self-reflectiveness, a self-questioning. And Heidegger realized, as we do, that not every person is moved to question herself or himself, to take an interrogative stance with regard to her or his condition or to the condition of the world. Simply accepting what is given, unable to imagine alternatives, too many passively accept or accede. It is at least conceivable that such persons cannot care (Heidegger, 1962, pp. 180–230).

Teachers and nurses, wishing to keep alive a dialogue of care with those with whom they work, need to keep their own questions alive and palpitant. That means existing in a dialectical relation to what is given, and summoning up imaginative visions of what might be, what ought to be (if, that is, things could be otherwise). The very notion of reaching toward open possibility is health-giving and empowering; therefore, imagination has much to do with care. We are situated beings, all of us, incomplete and in the making. We can see things and hear things only from our particular vantage points and against particular life stories; but, in our caring, we can try to make connections, to create metaphors, to bring about new fusions in our world.

Women's writings and women's novels render densely interwoven lives, touched by ambiguities, studded with passion, vibrant with desires to be. There are seldom either/ors. No matter what fictions I pick up— *The House of Mirth, The Dollmaker, Beloved, Tell Me a Riddle, The Good Mother*—there are relationships, sometimes sustaining, sometimes destructive. There are webs of relationship that release from rigid solitudes; there are webs that tangle and that bind. There are desires for stability and order; there is the nagging sense of things pulling apart or pulling down. It is in the midst of this, affirming our part in the human condition, that we heed the caring imperative. Let us acknowledge the tension and discover the passion. The spaces remain to be opened; care remains to be achieved.

REFERENCES

Alcoff, L. (1988). Cultural feminism versus post-structuralism: The identity crisis in feminist theory." In E. Minnich, J. O'Barr, & R. Rosenfeld (Eds.), *Reconstructing the academy: Women's education and women's studies.* Chicago: University of Chicago Press.

Arendt, H. (1961a). *Between past and future.* New York: Viking.

Arendt, H. (1961b). *Between past and future.* New York: Viking.

Arendt, H. (1972). *Crises of the republic.* New York: Harvest Books.

Belenkey, M. F. et al. (1987). *Women's ways of knowing.* New York: Basic Books.

Buber, M. (1957). *Between man and man.* New York: Dover.

Gilligan, C. (1981). *In a different voice.* Cambridge: Harvard University Press.

Heidegger, M. (1962). *Being and time.* New York: Harper & Row.

Kundera, M. (1984). *The unbearable lightness of being.* New York: Harper & Row.

Melville, H. (1986). Bartleby the scrivener. In *Billy Budd, sailor, and other stories by Herman Melville.* New York: Bantam.

Nietzsche, F. (1956). The genealogy of morals. In *The birth of tragedy and the genealogy of morals.* Garden City, NY: Doubleday Anchor.

Noddings, N. (1984). *Caring: A feminist ethic.* Berkeley: University of California Press.

Nussbaum, M. C. *The fragility of goodness: Luck and ethics in Greek tragedy and philosophy.* Cambridge: Cambridge University Press.

Schon, D. (1983). *The reflective practitioner.* New York: Basic Books.

Schutz, A. (1964). *Collected papers II. Studies in social theory.* The Hague: Martinus Nijhoff.

Stoppard, T. (1978). *Professional foul.* New York: Grove Press.

Walker, A. (1982). *The color purple.* New York: Washington Square Press.

Wolf, C. (1989). *Accident: A day's news.* New York: Farrar, Straus & Giroux.

Young-Bruehl, E. (1988). The education of women as philosophers. In E. Minnich, J. O'Barr, & R. Rosenfeld (Eds.), *Reconstructing the academy: Women's education and women's studies.* Chicago: University of Chicago Press.

4

Toward a Theory of Professional Nursing Caring: A Unifying Perspective

Dixie Koldjeski

The centrality of caring in nursing has long been recognized and provided as an essential aspect of professional practice. Although caring is universally associated with professional nursing, it continues to lack clarity in definition, description, meaning, structure, function, and healing qualities. Traditionally, caring has been linked to the nurturing and mothering role of women in society (Reverby, 1987). Brooks and Kleine-Kracht (1983) have shown that this role and the feminine gender connection have influenced the evolution of a definition of nursing over the decades.

The anchorage of caring in the powerful feminine image of caregiver has long contributed to confusion and difficulty in specifying differences between traditional caring and professional caring roles. A breakthrough was made in this respect by Leininger (1978, 1981) when she distinguished between generic caring, professional caring, and professional nursing care. The unified perspective here has been oriented by these definitions; however, a more comprehensive reformulation was undertaken to develop a paradigm for professional nursing caring.

The two major perspectives of caring developed by Leininger and Watson were selected as a starting point for the development of a more unified perspective (Leininger, 1978, 1980, 1981, 1984, 1988; Watson, 1979, 1985, 1988). Leininger has focused her research on identifying transcultural caring constructs in nursing and developing a nursing theory in which caring is the central focus. Watson's research has focused on the phenomenological and philosophical bases of caring, the development of carative factors using these perspectives, and the development of a theory emphasizing the philosophy and science of nursing caring (1985, 1988). In addition, views and questions expressed about caring and its survival have been considered (Carter, 1989; Kelly, 1988; Frye, 1985); a number of studies have also reported on perceptions of patients and nurses about caring and caring activities (Kahn & Steeves, 1988; Watson, 1988; Warren, 1988; Paternoster, 1988; Valentine, 1988; Larson, 1984; Gaut, 1983; Brown, 1982; Henry, 1975).

The two perspectives of caring developed by Leininger and Watson illuminate and connect particular aspects of nursing depending on the centrality each gives to philosophical, cultural, and empirical concerns. Each has different strengths and different emphases. For Leininger, caring is embedded in transcultural phenomena central to all of nursing; for Watson, caring has human dimensions that are embedded in an ethic and a moral ideal of human value accompanied by a commitment to preserve and restore the human center to nursing theory and practice. Guiding the unification process throughout is the view expressed by Colaizzi (1975) that the proper object of nursing science is the human experience of health and illness, that this experience is uniquely human and this fact places nursing within a dimension of reality that is different from technology.

In the unified perspective here, the interconnections between the humanistic, scientific, and experiential bases of caring and the unique aspects of professional nursing are central with an emphasis on unifying these aspects to identify a professional nursing caring paradigm. This paradigm has a structure that gives professional nursing caring both uniqueness and wholeness. The development of this paradigm has been a necessary first step in a quest to develop a nursing theory in which caring is systemically based. Such a theory would have additional organizing concepts, such as person-health related environments, energy force fields, and holistic nursing. Because of the importance of unifying many of the identified and significant aspects of caring, if they are to be theory-systemic, the unification process and the particular paradigm developed by this process are described.

The unified perspective owes much to many researchers, scholars, colleagues, graduate students, clinicians, clients, and patients. To these and to all theorists and researchers whose ideas and work have been studied and sometimes cited, a collective acknowledgment of their contributions to the advancement of the humanistic and scientific aspects of nursing caring is given.

ADVANCING THE SCIENCE OF PROFESSIONAL NURSING CARING

Concepts of caring have long guided and informed professional nursing practice and, more recently, research has begun to identify its nature and characteristics. This body of work has served as a base from which theory has advanced beyond an emphasis on concepts to one that promotes development and testing of different theoretical propositions woven from these concepts and related research.

The development of the unified perspective has proceeded in phases, the first of which included concept analysis, identification of recurring themes in the literature on caring, and consolidating major findings from research. Using this work as a major building block, a second phase consisted of reconceptualizing a framework comprehensive enough to accommodate major aspects of professional nursing caring, the metaparadigm of nursing, the holistic nursing perspective, energy and energy exchange, and professional nursing therapeutics.

Both Watson and Leininger have emphasized that caring must be embedded in the corpus of nursing theory so that it is an integral system. The unified perspective follows this principle and extends theory work further by: (1) consolidating the extensive number of caring concepts by retaining essential meanings but reducing overlaps; (2) reorganizing concepts and activities, irrespective of philosophical and theoretical bases, into two categories to reflect more clearly those that focused on humanistic qualities of caring and those that focused on traditional and scientific nursing actions considered integral to the competence aspects of caring; (3) distinguishing between the qualities, which have been called *essences,* and the nursing actions, which have been called *entities*; and (4) fusing the essences and entities to show how they are expressed through three holistic indicators—being, relating, and doing—that come together as a whole.

ASSUMPTIONS

Several major assumptions have guided the development of the unified perspective:

1. Professional nursing caring is central to nursing and has to be systematically embedded in paradigms and theories of nursing; all epiphenomena such theoretical statements address flow from this truth.

2. Professional nursing caring can unify two major world views, the totality and simultaneity paradigms (as identified by Parse, 1987), by which health and illness phenomena, life experiences, health-related environments and relationships, health technologies, and related therapeutics are commonly conceptualized by using general paradigms of reality to achieve wholeness and integration.

3. Professional nursing caring uses energy and energy exchange in general and focused ways through therapeutic use of self (nurse) to achieve healing and healthogenic outcomes as well as special kinds of illness outcomes in patient/client and nurse relationships.

4. Professional nursing caring occurs in various health-related environments and contexts, all of which interact with the actors and actions in these settings, thus influencing therapeutic use of self by nurses and the efficacy of nursing therapeutics.

5. Professional nursing caring has to be embedded in a professional socialization process that emphasizes both humanistic and scientific aspects of the therapeutic use of self.

REORGANIZATION OF CARING CONCEPTS

An early phase in the development of a more unified caring perspective was to conduct a critical analysis of a variety of caring concepts, caring factors, and caring activities to determine meanings with particular attention given to variations, similarities, and differences. This was done to reorganize them in a way that would retain original meanings but reduce them in number.

The reorganization of caring concepts fell into two categories: one that emphasized humanistic concepts and their meanings and importance in human experiences; the other focused on scientific and empiric factors of professional nursing. Although no preconceived number of concepts was considered for either category, the process yielded the 12 humanistic and 13 scientific concepts in Table 1.

Once reorganization of concepts had been completed, the next phase focused on translating the humanistic concepts to a basic core of unique qualities that seemed immanent in the concepts themselves and would represent the basic essences in professional nursing caring relationships.

Table 1

Humanistic Concepts	Scientific Concepts
Expressions of Feelings & Concern Through:	*Expression of Nursing Actions Through:*
Love	Helping
Faith	Sharing
Trust	Touching
Growth	Succoring
Empathy	Protecting
Presence	Supporting
Tenderness	Stimulating
Compassion	Decision making
Involvement	Health promotion
Hope instillment	Health maintenance
Self-actualization	Environmental restructuring
Interpersonal valuing	Maintaining human integrity
	Clinical judgments re technological monitoring

Five essences were identified as: *interpersonal valuing and involvement,* a valuation of person in terms of humanness and placing a premium on human needs, compassionate and sensitive care, and a willingness to become involved in these aspects of experiences as opposed to a focus on symptoms of disease and health technologies; *experiencing-with,* of *being-there,* actions and expressions based on an orientation consistent with "persons-as-beings" (Heidegger, 1962; Sartre, 1956), a position that assumes an ongoing personality process that is continuously open to change through actions, experiences, and feelings and in which opportunities are shaped for personal growth of both patient-client and nurse; *instillment of faith,* possibly hope, for whatever is to come, involves recognition and establishment of a need for harmony between spirit, soul, and reality; *concern and love for another,* the human need to be loved and cared for and about (Watson, 1985); and *actualization,* the use of energy through resonance (a principle of unitary life processes, Rogers, 1970), to facilitate the temporary merging of identities of patient-client and nurse to bring together intellect, emotions, and intuitions to enable a common sense of being-with, of being-there to develop through caring and then to formulate new energy patterns that promote healing and self-actualization for participants in such experiences.

For the scientific concepts, five entities involving independent nursing actions integral to existential reality in health and illness care were identified: *professional nursing relationships,* the special relations that use the core essences for focus, direction, and guide therapeutic use of self and include helping, sharing, touching, succoring, protecting, stimulating and supporting actions; *health promotion and maintenance* through health education and development and participation in actions that change noxious behaviors to more healthful behaviors; *nursing therapeutics,* the application of nursing science to wellness and illness processes, problems, and experiences; *environmental, contextual, and situational monitoring and restructuring* to create caring environments for both patients-clients and nurses; *maintaining human integrity (soma and psyche)* by incorporating the essences of caring in all nursing actions; and exercising clinical judgments associated with *technological management and monitoring* with compassionate consideration given to quality of living and a caring, loving, dying experience.

HOLOGRAPHIC PARADIGM OF REALITY

The next phase in developing the unified perspective was to select a general paradigm of reality in which concepts could be conceptualized to have a dynamic wholeness and structure of interconnections to the unique aspects of nursing. For this purpose, a holographic paradigm of reality (Boehm, 1985, 1980a, 1980b, 1978; Pribram, 1982; Ferguson, 1982; Weber, 1982; Wilbur, 1982) was used to structure caring concepts, relationships, and interconnections between the humanistic, scientific, and empirical bases of caring and the unique aspects of nursing. This general paradigm is unique in that it addresses the wholeness of reality for people, their experiences, health, and things.

The holographic paradigm posits that in any universe, each part of the universe is in the whole and the whole is in the part. In a universe, order and wholeness are achieved by two interconnecting realms: the *explicate realm,* where things and events are separate, unconnected, and have an unfolded order and the *implicate realm,* where things and events are undivided wholes. A key principle is that the implicate realm is available to the explicate realm, thus creating an enfolded order that has an inseparable interconnectedness between the two.

The holographic paradigm considers the nonlinear nature of reality. It focuses attention on seeking general themes and patterns when testing a particular model of reality by determining results by a first test and then repeating tests over time to discern small changes and variations. At some point, such changes become significant if enough transitions occur.

Ravn (1988) has elaborated on Boehm's paradigm by clarifying the characteristics and interconnections of the two different realms of reality. The implicate domain or the enfolded order (from Latin *plicare*, to fold) has little or no form and structure; there is no special locale for anything. Everything is everywhere, everything is folded into everything else, just as when an egg folded into a batter loses its separate and well-defined form and existence and is distributed throughout the batter. In contrast, in the explicate domain, or unfolded order, forms are distinguishable and occupy particular positions in space and time outside of each other and exist as entities. The implicate realm is a synonym for flux while the explicate realm is a synonym for form and structure for a particular order involving particular phenomena or systems. Since forms unfold spontaneously from flux, the implicate order generates creative power and energy from flux and human activity. This flux and activity in turn potentiates the generation and development of the explicate order involving form and substance.

Ravn believes that unfoldness and wholeness are not necessarily exclusive. Wholeness and unfoldness have positive value and, combined, create a reality that results in what Ravn calls a "holonomic order" (p. 102). Unfoldness without wholeness has negative value and is evident in differentiation, compartmentalization, and fragmentation. The unified perspective for professional nursing caring has used the holonomic order principle.

PROFESSIONAL NURSING CARING PARADIGM

The holographic paradigm of reality provided a general structure for the development of a holonomic order for a professional nursing caring paradigm. In the paradigm, holonomic order consists of the implicate realm of nursing where wholeness encompasses unique caring qualities —*the essences*. These are special kinds of nurse-patient relationships that are permeated with expressions of love, concern, and respect for another; of being-there available to exchange energies and communications; of experiencing-with another the humanness of life and death; of promoting self-actualization for other and self; of supporting and comforting in illness and death and in times of high vulnerability for other, moving to protect from harm's way and helping to mobilize personal, social, or carative resources.

In this holonomic order, the explicate realm consists of those relations, things, events, and realities—*the entities*—that are often unconnected and fragmented. They include health technologies that, while life-supporting or life-saving or both, become a focus in and of themselves; the influences of health-related environments on the human experience of illness and the situations and crises that characteristically arise; the situational contexts in which people find themselves in their search for and need of health care; the roles encompassed in nurse-patient relationships; the disconnected experiences and relationships that have few if any threads to weave them together in a pattern that has meaning for both the patient-client and the nurse; and the applications of various nursing and medical therapeutics that have a known structure and process designed to achieve a desired outcome(s) on some aspect of wellness and illness experiences.

The *interconnections* between the implicate realm in which the unique essences of professional caring are generated and energized and the explicate realm in which the entities are structured, initiated, and operationalized are the (1) holistic nursing perspective, (2) person-environment interactions in relation to wellness and illness, and (3) the caring ethic. As the essences and the entities interact through these special and dynamic unifying elements, *fusion* occurs, new order and energy are created and the whole is expressed through the holistic indicators of:

Being: presence, experiencing, actualizing, expressing compassion, concern, and love for other.

Relating: personally, interpersonally, and transpersonally.

Doing: professional nursing decisions and actions (nursing therapeutics).

These holistic indicators have embedded in their roles, structure, and functions the many meanings of caring in professional nursing. In fusion, the unification of the implicate and explicate orders, each of which has many different things in many different mixes, causes dynamic actions that generate an excess of energy and a different organization and structure for the things in the mix. This excess of energy and new organization becomes available to the professional nurse to

Table 2
Professional Nursing Caring Paradigm

IMPLICATE REALM of Essences (Unique Nursing Qualities)	is available to	EXPLICATE REALM of Entities (Professional Nursing Actions)
Actualization		Nursing therapeutics
Instillment of faith and hope		Restructuring of environments
Concern and love for another		Health promotion and maintenance
Experiencing—with and being there		Caring nurse-patient/client relationships
Interpersonal valuing and involvement		Maintaining human wholeness and integrity
		Technological management and monitoring

Essences and entities are particularized for professional nursing through interconnections

   □   The holistic nursing perspective

   □   Special kinds of person-environment health-related interactions

   □   The caring ethic

Fusion occurs when essences, entities, and interconnections become a whole (enfold) and expressed through the holistic indicators of:

Being: Presence, experiencing, compassion, actualization

Relating: Personally, interpersonally, transpersonally

Doing: Professional nursing caring actions

use in a more sustained and focused therapeutic use of self in healing and healthogenic actions. Table 2 is a representation of the professional nursing caring paradigm.

This paradigm of professional nursing caring has some similarity to the conceptualization of caring recently proposed by Benner and Werbel (1989). Using a philosophic perspective, these authors assert that the primary connection between nursing and curing and healing is caring. Further, caring is viewed as central to understanding human experiences of wellness and illness because it fuses thought, feeling, and action in giving and receiving help.

PROFESSIONAL NURSING CARING: .
THE IMPERATIVE

Nursing education is at a crossroads: one direction is a continuation of perspectives and curricula emphases that are grounded in the scientific method and essentially tied to medical disease models of illness; a second is a focus on the more subjective aspects of the health and illness experience; and a third is a fusion model addressing critical elements of these positions. The paradigm of professional nursing caring in which a fusion of essences and entities has been conceptually achieved addresses this latter position. The humanistic ideals and scientific goals of nursing can be unified into a whole and expressed through a special kind of relation involving being, relating, and doing.

The paradigm suggests that a definition of professional nursing caring could be: therapeutic use of self by nurse with patient through mutual participation in special kinds of relationships and interactions to effect changes in illness and health-related experiences that involve self, soma, and environments. The relationships, interactions, and actions are special in the sense of their mix of scientific and humanistic knowledge bases, constancy and intensity of expressions of compassion, love, and hope; of maintaining integrity and actualization of body, self, and spirit; and the extent to which nursing actions are embedded in these essences and executed with knowledge and competence.

The imperative in nursing is that educators become more sensitized to how professional nursing caring is being conceptualized, taught, and practiced in nursing education curricula. There has perhaps been an overreliance on the so-called scientific process, translated as "the nursing process," in terms of expecting problem-solving based on linearity, rationality, and observability of phenomena to encompass much of the human experience in health and illness. In effect, the nursing process tends to purge feelings and phenomena not congruent with its basic scientific assumptions. The redeeming grace is that experienced nurses go beyond phenomena generated by use of the nursing process and use their professional sense and judgment to address the more humanistic aspects of people's experiences and to care.

The major challenge facing nursing today is to incorporate professional nursing caring in nursing curricula as its systemic dynamism. It is little wonder that this notion has been called revolutionary for it will involve new perspectives and knowledge, different kinds of role-modeling by faculty for students, different practice models, restructuring of nursing environments, and a deeper understanding of the healing properties of caring. A part of this understanding concerns the nature of professional nursing caring: not all care is provided in a transpersonal context of caring; not all care is directed toward a person but toward activities and technology; not all caring uses the energy generated through fusion in professional nursing caring to assist healthogenic changes to occur in health and illness experiences of patients-clients.

SUMMARY

This paradigm of professional nursing caring unifies aspects of humanistic and scientific perspectives. Through interconnections of the holistic nursing perspective, person-environment interactions, and the caring ethic, fusion occurs that reorganizes old orders and structures. From this dynamic, creative energies are generated and used in being, relating, and acting by the nurse through therapeutic use of self. Through professional nursing caring, the wholeness and integrity of a patient-client is maintained and assisted toward actualization, with wellness and illness outcomes altered, and more caring health-related environments restructured that preserve and support the humanness of patients and people in those environments.

The professional nursing paradigm has been guided in organization by a holographic perspective of reality, a perspective that envisions two realms: the implicate and the explicate, with the implicate available to the explicate realm in dealing with reality. The two realities have been unified into a holonomic order in which the essences (qualities) and entities (actions) of professional nursing caring have been restructured into a new order. The paradigm opens avenues for constructing a nursing theory in which caring is systematically embedded in concepts, structure, and relations.

The imperative for nursing education is to reconceptualize professional nursing caring and undertake the effort and energy required to place this essence in the heart of nursing theory, practice, education, and research. This is the profession's challenge for the coming decade.

REFERENCES

Benner, P., & Wrubel, J. (1989). *The primacy of caring.* Menlo Park, CA: Addison-Wesley.

Boehm, D. (1978). The enfolding-unfolding universe. *Revision: A Journal of Knowledge and Consciousness, 1,* 24–25.

Boehm, D. (1980a). *Wholeness and the implicate order.* London: Routledge & Kegan Paul.

Boehm, D. (1980b). The enfolded order and consciousness. In G. Epstein (Ed.), Studies in nondeterministic psychology. New York: Human Sciences Press.

Boehm, D. (1985). Fragmentation and wholeness in religion and science. *Zygon, 20*(1), 125–134.

Brooks, J. A., & Kleine-Kracht, A. E. (1983). Evolution of a definition of nursing. *Advances in Nursing Science, 5*(4), 51–58.

Carter, M. A. (1989). Professional practice: Why do we care? *Journal of Professional Nursing, 5*(2), 65.

Colaizzi, J. (1975). The proper object of nursing science. *International Journal of Nursing Studies, 12,* 197–200.

Ferguson, M. (1982). Karl Pribram's changing reality. In K. Wilbur (Ed.), *The holographic paradigm and other paradoxes.* Boulder, CO: Shambala.

Fry, S. (1988). The ethic of caring: Can it survive nursing? *Nursing Outlook, 36*(1), 48.

Gaut, D. A. (1984). Development of a theoretically adequate description of caring. *Western Journal of Nursing Research, 5*(4), 313–324.

Heidegger, M. (1962). *Being and time* (J. Macquarrie and E. S. Robinson, Trans.). New York: Harper & Row.

Henry, D. M. (1975). Nurse behaviors perceived by patients as indicators of caring. *Dissertation Abstracts International, 36,* 02–652B.

Kahn, D. L., & Steeves, R. H. (1988). Caring and practice: Construction of the nurse's world. *Scholarly Inquiry for Nursing Practice, 2*(3), 201–216.

Kelly, L. (1988). Editorial: The ethic of caring: Has it been discarded? *Nursing Outlook, 36*(1), 17.

Larson, P. (1984). Important nurse caring behaviors perceived by subjects with cancer. *Oncology Nursing Forum, 11*(6) 46–50.

Leininger, M. M. (1978). *Transcultural nursing concepts, theories, and practices.* New York: Wiley.

Leininger, M. M. (1980). Caring: A central focus of nursing and health care. *Nursing and Health Care, 1*(3), 135–143.

Leininger, M. M. (1981). The phenomenon of caring: Importance, research questions and theoretical considerations. In M. Leininger (Ed.), *Caring: An essential human need.* Thorofare, NJ: Slack.

Leininger, M. M. (1984). Care: The essence of nursing and health care. In M. M. Leininger (Ed.), *Care: The essence of nursing and health care.* Thorofare, NJ: Slack.

Leininger, M. M. (1988). Leininger's theory of nursing: Cultural care diversity and universality. *Nursing Science Quarterly, 1* (4), 152–160.

Parse, R. R. (1987). Paradigms and theories. In R. R. Parse (Ed.), *Nursing science: Major paradigms, theories, and critiques.* Philadelphia: Saunders.

Paternoster, J. (1988). How patients know that nurses care about them. *Journal of the New York State Nurses Association, 19*(4), 17–21.

Pribram, K. H. (1982). What the fuss is all about. In K. Wilbur (Ed.), *The holographic paradigm and other paradoxes.* Boulder, CO: Shambala.

Ravn, I. (1988). Holonomy: An ethic of wholeness. *Journal of Humanistic Psychology, 28*(3), 98–118.

Reverby, S. (1987). A caring dilemma: Womanhood and nursing in historical perspective. *Nursing Research, 36*(1), 5–11.

Rogers, M. (1970). *The theoretical basis of nursing.* Philadelphia: Davis.

Sartre, J. P. (1956). *Being and nothingness.* (H. Barnes, Trans.). New York: Philosophical Library.

Valentine, L. D. (1988). History, analysis, and application of the carative tradition in health and nursing. *Journal of the New York State Nurses Association, 19*(4), 4–9.

Warren, L. D. (1988). Review and synthesis of nine nursing studies on care and caring. *Journal of the New York State Nurses Association, 19*(4), 10–16.

Watson, J. (1979). *Nursing: The philosophy and science of caring.* Boston: Little, Brown.

Watson, J. (1985). *Nursing: Human science and human care.* Norwalk, CT: Appleton-Century-Crofts.

Watson, J. (1988). New dimensions of human caring theory. *Nursing Science Quarterly, 1*(4), 175–181.

Weber, R. (1982). The enfolding-unfolding universe: A conversation with David Boehm. In K. Wilbur (Ed.), *The holographic paradigm and other paradoxes.* Boulder, CO: Shambala.

Wilbur, K. (1982). (Ed.), *The holographic paradigm and other paradoxes.* Boulder, CO: Shambala.

5

Dependent and Authentic Care: Implications of Heidegger for Nursing Care

John R. Scudder, Jr.

Heidegger's treatment of care can make two important contributions to understanding nursing care. The first concerns the way in which care is given and can either make patients dependent or self-directing. Second, Heidegger helps us to see how each type of care is related to our being and becoming.

Heidegger describes two ways of caring. In the first way, a person will "leap in" for another and "take over for the other." This form of care can readily foster domination and dependency when the caregiver "leaps in and takes away 'care.'" I will call the latter dependent care because it fosters dependency on others. In contrast to dependent care, authentic care (so named by Heidegger) occurs when the caregiver will "leap ahead [*ihm vorausspringt*] in his existential potentiality-for-being, not in order to take away his 'care' but rather to give it back to him authentically" (Heidegger, 1972, pp. 159–160). Thus, in authentic care, the other is helped to care for his own being.

Heidegger helps us to understand that these two forms of caring are essential aspects of human being and becoming. Care (*Sorge*) is for Heidegger an essential, if not the essential, existential of human being.

By existential, he means that which refers to human being and becoming, as opposed to the characteristics of things. He believes that Western language has forced thinking about humans into categories that are more appropriate for thinking about things rather than human beings.

For Heidegger, care is that which unifies actuality and possibility (Gelven, 1970, p. 74). All things exist at the level of actuality in that their being is determined by other forces. Even the higher mammals that seem to care for each other do so on the basis of some combination of genetics and conditioning. Human beings are those beings who can care for their own being because they can recognize and fulfill possibilities in their actual situation. For Heidegger, freedom means to act to fulfill possibilities that are present in our actual situation. Since humans are capable of recognizing possibilities in their actual situation and have the ability, within limits, to realize them, they are beings who can choose their own being by caring for their being.

Obviously for Heidegger, care is focused on future possibility and on freedom. Usually, when most Westerners think of care, they think of actuality rather than possibility and of beneficient control rather than freedom. It is easy to see why care is thought of as actuality and control when one examines health care. After all, those who must seek help from medical and nursing experts are dependent on them for their well-being. All nurses have given extreme forms of dependent care, when patients are completely unable to care for themselves. They have seen the gratitude in patients' eyes for care given. But they have also seen the frustration, the despair, and the hatred in the eyes of very self-directed persons who now have to be waited on hand and foot, as a result of serious illness. Nurses know both of the dependency of those receiving health care and of their desire for self-care.

Nurses also know that all nursing care is necessarily related to possibility. Nursing care is given in the hope of fostering possible well-being. Having to care for someone when there is absolutely no hope fosters despair. This is why the Karen Ann Quinlan case remains so prominent in our thoughts. When actuality rules out possibility, care loses its primary meaning.

For Heidegger, the relationship of actuality and possibility is one of time. He develops this analysis of care in *Being and Time* (1972), in which he argues that the primary essence of man is "being in time." His interpretation of time, often called lived time, means pushing toward a projected future drawing on the past and making choices in the present that actualize future possibilities. Put differently, being in time means being directed toward possibilities that grow out of actuality, the fulfillment of which requires drawing on an actual past so as to bring about present action which attempts to fulfill projected future possibilities of being.

When future possibilities, past actualities, and present action relate to each other harmoniously, this is called *coherence in time*. For example, some patients willingly choose therapy that involves enduring more pain if this means they will recover more rapidly and will be able to leave the hospital sooner and resume their normal lives. The possibility of resuming normal life calls forth the resources necessary to endure the short-term pain required for therapeutic action which enhances the possibility of resuming a normal life. In contrast, several nurses in a study (Bishop & Scudder, in press) conducted on fulfillment in nursing in a tertiary medical center reported that their most unfulfilling moment as nurses was when their patients who had literally no hope of recovery were subjected to countless interventions that made the remainder of their lives painful and miserable in an attempt to keep them biologically alive without regard for the quality of that life. Indeed, one sensed that these nurses felt that such medical care was dictated by the needs of the physician to give medical care rather than the desire to help the patient live the best possible life for the remainder of his or her life. Also, in such cases, what the patient desired often was not considered unless one regards signing a consent form as adequate consideration of how one would want to live the remainder of his or her life given the present situation and the possibilities for treatment. Considerations of coherence in time are extremely important in health care because health care is aimed at better possible well-being, the accomplishment of which concerns the actual condition of the patient, the abilities and resources of health care workers, and the formulation and execution of a plan of action that fosters the well-being of the patient in ways which are in accord with his or her understanding of the good life. When these actualities and possibilities make sense as a whole, then coherence in time is achieved, which, if we follow Heidegger, actually means that good health *care* is being given.

Although Heidegger asserts the primacy of possibility over actuality, he regards both as essential. For Heidegger, one is thrown into the world and initially does not choose his or her actuality—for example, parents, time of life, societal situations, size, sex, or health potential. Most persons do not choose to become ill, even those who contribute to their illness by engaging in such activities as excessive smoking, eating, or drinking. Whatever the cause, their illness is experienced as an actuality that affects their whole being. Their ability to project themselves into the future is temporarily or permanently altered. Sometimes those giving health care, especially physicians, fail to recognize this in their zeal to regard illness as a taxonomic category and subsume the person under the diagnostic category. This kind of thinking fails to recognize how deeply illness does affect persons. If we follow Heidegger, the patient's actuality is not the disease objectified and categorized but rather what the person with the illness is experiencing.

Alsop (1973) made this very evident in commenting on his own way of being during the serious illness that eventually led to his death. He pointed out that most people think of death from the perspective of wellness, but when human being was diminished to the degree that he had experienced it, death looked very different. Patients face death with despair, resignation, and sometimes even with a sense of relief. Heidegger recognizes this human way of being as the moods which constitute human actuality. Thus, the actuality of the patient who has given up is not the fact that the patient has incurable cancer and is being treated palliatively but that the patient lives in despair.

Living in despair is the actuality within which the nurse who cares for that patient must help him or her find possibilities. After all, the medical prognosis is not what the patient experiences, but despair is. Nurses would regard despair as the patient's response to illness if they followed the American Nurses' Association's (ANA) definition of nursing as "diagnosis and treatment of human responses to actual or potential health problems" (1980). In contrast, Heidegger would say that the patient's way of being is despair. Those nurses who follow the ANA's definition might say that responding to terminal or permanently disabling disease with despair is a way of being. But how we phrase this response and propose to care for the despairing person indicates whether or not we regard it as a way of being. For example, if it is a way of being, we would not say that one responded *with* despair but that one was *in* despair. After all, responding with despair is very different from being in despair. When the actuality for a patient is to be severely disabled for the rest of his or her relatively short life, whatever possibility for hope of a better life must be found within these actualities.

An example of despair is given by Zaner in an excerpt of a tape recording from a patient.

> Well, here's *another* day. . . . I'll swear, how slowly they pass . . . and you wonder why I can't be cheerful about things. . . . I'm trying, I really am tryin', but I'm not gettin' anywhere. . . . When he [her pulmonary specialist] told me that there wasn't any possible chance for me to get out and have another apartment on my

own . . . and . . . that I'd always have to live in a place like this
. . . that . . . that did somethin' to me. . . . I really couldn't
shake it. . . . I know I'm gloomy and sad, an' all that. You'll just
have to bear with me. . . . I may get used to it, an' I may not . . .
'ts a bad deal. . . . (1988, p. 268).

Obviously, those who were caring for this patient had conveyed to her
that she should be happy. After all, she only faces the actuality of living
the rest of her life in a place and situation that she finds intolerable. If
her nurses are to help her find possibilities and hence hope, they must
do so by helping her discover and realize the possibilities within her
actual situation of being ill in the nursing home.

Her problem is not merely the consequence of her illness but also the
result of the kind of nursing care she is receiving, as she makes very clear.

I know . . . I know that no matter . . . how long my sentence is
. . . it's gonna be spent in a nursing home, alone. . . . Can't think
of a worse way to spend it th' . . . than in a nursing home. Which is
just like bein' in jail, really. You have no rights; you're just a number. A baby. An' all the bodies are old and worn out, an' yours is no
different than anybody else's. . . . An' I found that it's not any
advantage at all . . . to have your . . . brains left, because, when
you question things, they think you're trying to tell them how to run
their business. . . . It's better not to question, it's better just t' go
'n accept their discipline like a child would (1988, p. 268).

Obviously, one reason she feels sentenced is that she is having self-care
taken from her. Facing the remainder of one's life in a nursing home
away from one's family is depressing enough without having to deny that
you've "got brains." Obviously, the first step in giving authentic care
would be to allow the patient to use her brains in assuming the maximum
possible self-direction. In this case, recognizing that the patient has
brains and the ability to make her own decisions might be enough to help
her begin to see the possibilities for living in the nursing home for the
remainder of her life.

Being made dependent is abhorrent to this patient. She is a self-
directing person who equates losing self-care to a prison sentence. The
patient, although deeply in despair, is obviously not willing to turn her
brains over to others. She wants to direct her own life but finds that
impossible because she is given the same dependent care as those who
have no brains. A person who lives in despair cannot see possibilities for
better life. Consequently, it isn't likely that such a person will care for

him or herself. Thus, willingness to care for self involves seeing possibilities which give hope.

Recognition of possibilities must, of course, take seriously the actuality. For example, the possibilities for a person with a fast-progressing terminal illness are set within the context of a short life expectancy. Their willingness to care for themselves is related to the possibilities they see within this context. One positive example of realizing limited possibilities in the face of a terminal illness was shared by a senior nursing student in a study on fulfillment in nursing: "As a nursing student I was assigned to a dying patient. In the midst of all her pain and suffering, she constantly praised everything I did for her. Just to experience the presence of a person so at peace with herself was a terrific highlight in my life" (Scudder & Bishop, 1986, p. 148). Obviously, this patient not only realized the possibilities for living well within the actuality of a short life expectancy but also helped her nursing student to recognize the possibilities of being a good nurse and a fine human being.

All patient care is founded on seeing possibilities for fostering patient well-being. These possibilities can range from full recovery to limiting the pain in the face of certain and painful death. In any case, the nurse's actual care of the patient grows out of the possibility she sees for better patient well-being. The crucial question concerns whether or not the nurse focuses the possibilities of care on the patient's self-care. Obviously, there are situations in which the nurse must stress taking care of patients. Immediately after major surgery a patient obviously cannot climb out of bed to use the toilet. In such cases the nurse's care of that patient grows out of an ability to recognize how his or her actions will enhance the possibility of patient well-being. But when the nurse literally takes care of the patient, this should imply that the patient is unable to take care of him or herself. We all know nurses sometimes care for their patients out of their own need to care. This laudable need to care for others hides a real danger, however. It is easy for the *need* to care to blind one to the possibilities for self-care. When this occurs, the nurse rather than taking care *of* the patient is actually taking care *from* the patient. When nurses take care *from* the patient, they deny the patient the possibility of self-care that is essential to being fully human.

When nurses take care *of* patients rather than taking care *from* patients, they fulfill the moral sense of nursing by fostering the well-being of patients. The moral sense of nursing asserts the priority of possibility over actuality that, for Heidegger, leads to being authentic. Inauthentic human beings give priority to actuality over possibility in that they let their past self or others (*das man*) dictate their actions and therefore their way of being in the world. In contrast, an authentic person chooses his or her own life from the possibilities present in the world. An inauthentic nurse would let others take caregiving *from* him or her by following past teachers of nursing, supervisors, procedure manuals, peer pressure, and even his or her own past self. An authentic nurse would choose a unique way of caring for each particular patient. This, of course, does not imply inventing nursing practice anew with each patient. Instead, he or she would appropriate sound nursing practice into his or her own way of being as a nurse. Care would be creatively given in response to particular patients for whom the nurse assumes responsibility.

The contention that nurses ought to give authentic care obviously states a moral imperative, even though Heidegger himself did not interpret authenticity and inauthenticity as moral issues. Indeed, the possibility of developing a Heideggerian ethic is a major problem for interpreters of Heidegger. Heidegger does, however, point ethics in the right direction by asserting the priority of possibility over actuality. After all, morality deals with what ought to be. What ought to be is what is actually not now but could be and should be. The practice of nursing itself is founded on the moral imperative that people ought to be well. Nursing practice consists of ways of fostering the physical and psychological well-being of persons. When illness or debilitation make persons incapable of caring for their own well-being, they rely on the expert care of nurses. Such care fosters dependence when the nursing care given takes care *from* them. Taking care *of* them when they are unable to care for themselves is not taking care *from* them. But when this dependent relationship prevents patients from recognizing and achieving self-care, then care for their being is taken *from* them.

CONCLUSION

Heidegger's philosophy of care has led us to interpret the meaning of nursing care within the broader context of what it means to be human. He has helped us to see that nursing is not only founded on care but that care can inhibit as well as enhance human well-being. The fact that the ill need help in recognizing and fulfilling their possibilities makes them dependent on others. Authentic nurses work to make those for whom they care free from dependency. However, nurses often work with those who will never be free of nursing care. But even in these cases, they should seek to minimize dependent care and maximize authentic care.

The ill, after all, are like the well in that their capacity for authentic living is related to the possibilities inherent in their situation. They are different from the well in that illness and debilitation have temporarily or permanently limited these possibilities. Nursing care becomes authentic care when nurses give responding and responsible care that enhances, restores, or increases self-care to the degree possible. By so doing, patients are not merely helped to cope with illness and debilitation but are encouraged and empowered to continue their quest for full humanity.

REFERENCES

Alsop, Stewart. (1973). *Stay of execution: A sort of memoir.* Philadelphia: Lippincott.

American Nurses' Association. (1980). *Nursing: A social policy statement.* Kansas City, MO: American Nurses' Association.

Bishop, A., & Scudder, J. R., Jr. (In press). *The practical, moral and personal sense of nursing: A phenomenological philosophy of practice.* Albany, NY: State University of New York Press.

Gelven, M. (1970). *A commentary on Heidegger's "Being and Time."* New York: Harper.

Heidegger, M. (1972). *Being and time* (J. Macquarrie & E. Robinson, Trans.). New York: Harper & Row. (Original work published 1927).

Scudder, J. R., Jr., & Bishop, A. H. (1986). The moral sense and health care. In A-T. Tymieniecka (Ed.), *Moral sense in the communal significance of life. Analecta Husserliana 20* (pp. 125–158). Dordrecht-Boston: D. Reidel.

Zaner, R. M. (1988). *Ethics and the clinical encounter.* Englewood Cliffs, NJ: Prentice-Hall.

6

Nursing Education as
Authentic Nursing Care

Anne H. Bishop

The primary implication of Heidegger's two forms of care discussed by Scudder is that nurses should not take care from patients but should help patients learn to care for themselves as much as possible. The first form of care Heidegger describes as that in which a person will "leap in" for another and "take over for the Other" (1972, p. 158). Nurses will recognize the many instances where they must leap in and take over from the other. Patients who are unconscious, burned, in traction, or too weak to give their own care are among those for whom nurses must take over the care. Nurses also often have to take over the care of patients because the patient's condition might be compromised if they were to exert too much effort—for example, patients with a massive myocardial infarction or those with chronic obstructive pulmonary disease. But this form of care can foster domination and dependency when the caregiver "leaps in and takes away 'care.'"

The most obvious form of this type of care is when the nurse acts out of a desire to dominate as exemplified by the "big nurse" in *One Flew Over the Cuckoo's Nest* (Kesey, 1973). But I doubt that most nurses are motivated mainly by the desire to dominate. More often they take care from patients in subtle and unrecognized ways. The nature of nursing care fosters dependent care on both sides. When patients become accustomed to being cared for by nurses, they may be reluctant to assume responsibility for their own care. Nurses become accustomed to caring for patients and experiencing the gratitude of dependent persons for the good care they have received. Examples in which care is taken from patients subtly and usually unknowingly are when nurses:

1. Proceed to give the care themselves to avoid a confrontation with patients who are reluctant to assume their own care.
2. Speak to a family member or the patient's physician for patients rather than paving the way and supporting patients in their own communication.
3. Fail to give patients sufficient information to care for self (inadequate patient teaching and discharge planning).

Regardless of whether care is taken away from the desire to dominate or is simply eroded, when nurses take care away the patient is made dependent on the nurse. Such dependency undermines the patient's ability for self-care and, in so doing, lessens his humanity.

The second form of care that Heidegger describes is that in which the caregiver will "leap ahead" [*ihm vorausspringt*] in his existential potentiality-for-being, not to take away his 'care' but rather to give it back to him authentically" (1972, pp. 158–159). Thus, the person is helped to care for his or her own being. Nurses who practice so that they give care back to patients authentically will be preoccupied, in Ortega's sense (1960), with fostering a patient's ability to care for self. Fostering self-care requires discussing with the patient what he or she views as his or her capabilities; determining what the patient needs to know about the illness or hospitalization to make self-care possible; and ensuring that the patient assumes only that level of self-care that is within his or her possibilities.

Nursing education seems to prepare nursing students for both taking care of patients and fostering authentic self-care. Most beginning courses in nursing education programs teach students the skills necessary for taking care of patients by having them learn such fundamental skills as personal hygiene and mobility. All nursing education programs probably provide some opportunities for students to participate in the care of patients restricted by coma, surgery, casts, traction, burns, or other such immobilizing situations. However, nursing educators also foster self-care by stressing patient teaching, early ambulation, and early discharge. And, of course, self-care is supported by some theories of nursing, especially that of Dorothea Orem (1980). However, the crucial issue, if we follow Heidegger, is not the skills taught or the theory used, but whether or not students are taught to help patients recognize their possibilities for self-care and to empower them to fulfill those possibilities.

I will argue that nursing education inadequately prepares students to deal with patient possibilities because first, it stresses the sciences and practical know-how to the neglect of the humanities; second, it stresses disease rather than illness; and third, it stresses the professional world of the nurse to the neglect of the lived world of the patient and direct personal communication with the patient. Put positively, education for authentic care requires greater emphasis on the humanities, on the experience of illness, and on communicating with patients concerning their lived world.

First, nursing education, by stressing the sciences and neglecting the humanities, inclines nurses to look for theoretical prescriptions rather than for possibilities to be realized. The effect of such an education was evident in the answer given by a very successful electronics inventor when asked how he had become so successful when his formal education stressed philosophy and neglected science and technology. He answered that the study of science and technology inclines one to follow the dictates of theory, whereas the study of philosophy emphasized looking for new possibilities. Of course, science can be taught creatively and philosophy prescriptively, but the point here is that science focuses on what is and the humanities on what could be and ought to be.

The prescriptive thought of scientific knowledge and research methods has influenced the language and thought of nurses concerning human beings. We often find references in the nursing literature to adaptation and to internal and external environments and their influence on the behavior of humans. The language we use to talk about such adaptation is largely a result of social science research that has copied the hard sciences and has viewed the human being as an organism which only reacts to external force. Such thinking reduces the richness of our existence by neglecting what it is possible for us to become.

What type of curriculum would emphasize a person's ability to choose from among possibilities? How can we help students to recognize possibilities in their practice and foster self-care of their patients? Students would first need to have an understanding of what it means to be human, what it means to be well, and what it means to be ill. A foundation in philosophy and the humanities is essential for this knowledge. While nursing education has prided itself on expanding the curriculum in our collegiate programs, all too often that expansion occurs in areas of sociology and psychology that have modeled themselves after the basic sciences. The result of this modeling has led to the development of behavioral sciences and research that treats humans as any organism. Consequently, the language of the behavioral sciences has become prevalent in many nursing education programs. An alternative to such research is the study of groups or individuals from a human science approach, which treats humans as subjects rather than objects and begins with the lived experience of persons. I fear that in our quest to make nursing more scientific and to find prescriptive theories of nursing and in our zeal to copy the language of diagnosis of our physician colleagues, nursing may be limiting the options that we make available to patients for their care, thereby taking away the very human characteristic of our ability to choose.

Certainly, students must know much of the scientific material that is currently in the nursing curriculum. It would be impossible for nurses to work as full members of the health care team if they did not understand the language of medicine. When the physician writes a medical diagnosis on a patient's chart, nurses already have some understanding of the physiological changes that are taking place in the patient's body. The advancement of medical science has given health care professionals knowledge about the actualities of bodily processes when a patient has a particular diagnosis. But diagnosis names the disease to be treated, not the patient's illness that is experienced.

What patients experience, however, is not a disease but an illness that disrupts their lived world. Rawlinson (1982) describes illness as a rupture in the man-world relationship:

> Illness names that experience in which our own everyday embodied capacities fail us. Illness obstructs our ordinary access to the world and presents the body as a signifier for the way in which we are limited and can be impeded in our encounter with the world (p. 74).

She contends that illness alters this man-world relationship in four ways. First, the body becomes the center of our concerns and fills our consciousness almost in direct proportion to the severity of our illness. Second, our body seems unreliable and unpredictable. We are not able to depend on our embodiment in our usual ways. Tasks that have been second nature to us are no longer possible or must be altered in some way. Third, we realize in illness that we are not merely determined by our own choosing. We become acutely aware of our own finiteness and of our possible or actual loss of self. Fourth, "illness distorts our ordinary relationship with others insofar as it debilitates, humiliates, and isolates" (1982, pp. 75–76).

To understand the lived world of patients, students must learn to listen and communicate with empathy about the patient's experience of illness. One example of entering into the patient's experience is given in Hasting's discussion with a patient of how she had experienced rheumatoid arthritis.

> I then moved into doing a physical assessment and looking at her various joints. Thinking about this later, I realized one of the ways I was able to communicate with her, really get to some of the things she felt, was just by the *way* I looked at her joints. I made distinctions about the swelling, the level of inflammation, and so on. It is possible to touch a person and move the person's hand or wrist, and say: "I can tell that this must be really painful right now," or "It looks like you haven't been able to use this hand for a long time," or "What is this finger doing way out here? This must be really difficult when you take a bath."
>
> She said: "You know, no one has even talked about it as a personal thing before, no one's ever talked to me as if this were a thing that mattered, a personal event" (Benner & Wrubel, 1989, pp. 10–11).

Another nurse had so entered into the experience of her patients who had had mastectomies that one patient at the end of her preoperative teaching on mastectomy could not believe that the nurse had not had a mastectomy herself (Benner & Wrubel, 1989, p. 13). Student nurses need to learn to enter into their patient's experience of illness, which, after all, is the actuality that confronts the patient.

When nurses enter into the experience of patients, they have entered their lived world. Although their illness tends to become focal, their lived world involves much more. If nurses are to help patients realize their possibilities for a better life, they must enter the patient's lived world, as is evident in the following example from our study of fulfillment in nursing. One nurse who had given care for nearly a year to a 25-year-old woman with third-degree burns over 60% of her body stated:

> I spent an average of three to four hours per day carrying out the doctor's orders as well as providing essential nursing care. We came to know each other as I have never known another patient. She trusted me and talked of her husband's alcoholism, her concern for the welfare and safety of three small children, financial worries and her physical pain and depression (Scudder & Bishop, 1986, p. 145).

Another nurse in our study related:

> Two years ago I had the opportunity to deliver total patient care to a
> 25-year-old girl with end-stage congestive cardiomyopathy. She was
> in congestive heart failure with many ventricular life-threatening
> arrhythmias. She was well aware of the fact that she was going to die
> and admitted her fright to me and also asked me point blank if she
> was going to die. We were able to discuss such problems as how could
> this be explained to her 7-year-old daughter? Who would care for her
> 7-year-old daughter and her own 16-year-old retarded sister? I also
> discussed with her family some of the fears she had acknowledged
> and encouraged them to discuss these things with her (Scudder &
> Bishop, 1986, pp. 146–147).

Another nurse was able to communicate so openly with her patient about
her impending death that she could say, "We cried together, laughed
together, and conspired together to meet her needs even if it meant
bending hospital policy" (Scudder & Bishop, 1986, p. 149).

   In these examples, the nurses openly communicated with patients
about so-called private aspects of their lives. Recent talk about patients'
rights has inclined many students to avoid dealing with private matters,
but choosing possibilities usually involves discussing personal matters.
The right to privacy means that a nurse, simply by virtue of being a
nurse, does not have the right to deal with personal matters uninvited.
But students often need help in learning how to communicate with
patients in ways that invite personal discussion concerning possibilities
related to their care and recovery.

   How do nursing educators help students engage in personal conversations with patients concerning possibilities for self-care? Certainly, nursing educators recognize the importance of communication for nurses.
However, communication is often taught from a theoretical approach
and with an assumption that there is only one way to communicate that
will elicit the response desired from patients. A strategy that I recently
used in teaching a psychiatric-mental health nursing course had the
unexpected consequence of helping students to see numerous possibilities in communicating with their patients. Like many other courses in
psychiatric-mental health nursing, students use process recordings to
enhance their communication skills. A process recording requires the
student to record both the student's and the client's statements. The
assignment is then used for a variety of experiences, including evaluating
how the student is communicating in response to the client and in determining student values that influence the communication.

Although process recordings are most often used in a one-to-one evaluation between student and instructor, I recently experimented by using process recordings in a group setting with students. The first part of the semester, I used the process recordings in individual student conferences, but toward the end of the semester when the students were more comfortable with the psychiatric setting and trusted each other, I read aloud several interactions between a student and a client. I did not identify the student who had completed the interaction, but the students usually admitted who had done the process recording. After reading the student's response to the client, I asked the other students how they would interpret the student's response if they were the client and what response they would have made had they been talking with the client. Students were often able to give multiple interpretations and to provide a more appropriate response. The students indicated that this was a learning experience that helped them get in touch with their own values and see the possibilities available to develop more open communication with their clients. The sharing of process recordings also helped the students to see blocks in communication created by certain nurse responses. While I did not intentionally use this sharing technique as an implementation of Heidegger's possibilities, it certainly did assist students to consider the various possibilities available in open communication with clients.

While nursing educators recognize that helping students to communicate effectively is basic to all nursing care, one of the most difficult nursing situations is that in which the patient is experiencing despair because of a terminal illness or a deteriorating physical condition. A recent filmstrip, "Hopelessness" (Concept Media, 1989), gives suggestions for helping a patient to lessen his or her despair. The suggestions include acknowledging the patient's feelings of hopelessness, helping the patient to see he or she has someone to live for, and helping the patient to focus on those who are close to him or her. Each of these suggestions starts with the significant meanings that the patient has shared with his nurse. Significant meanings require the nurse to develop a personal relationship with the patient and to be willing to discuss the importance of others to the patient. For students to develop this kind of personal relationship with a patient requires that they have opportunities to know some patients over time and that they care for patients who are in despair. The emphasis in these nursing practice opportunities must be on knowing the patient and being open to the patient's concerns about the lived world. Finding such learning opportunities for students is more difficult with the prevalence of short hospital stays. However, having a student visit a patient with a long-term or terminal illness for an hour every week or two during a semester can be a valuable experience in helping students understand the patient's perspective from the lived world.

Another way in which students can learn to help patients consider possibilities is to give students the opportunity to be creative in planning for the patient's care. While the nursing process has sharpened our view of nursing's responsibilities for care of the patient, there is always the danger that the nursing process will be organized methodologically so that the options for care are limited. Teachers of nursing often expect students to come up with one perfect plan that fits the prescriptions of the health care community.

While the nursing process stresses ongoing evaluation and revision of the plan if it is not working, I wonder why we don't discuss with patients at the outset the options that are available with an explanation of why one may be preferable to another. Such communication of the priorities for care as seen from the nursing perspective could allow the patient to match the priorities with his or her own life-world possibilities. Such authentic planning between patient and nurse would overcome the impression, often given when we talk about patient noncompliance, of only *one* possibility of care. If patients were involved in their own care, they would realize what Zaner (1985) contends that every patient wants to know, namely, that those "who care for them *really* care" (p. 92). Not only that, but they would become responsible for participating in their own care. As one patient, a heart attack victim, expressed it, "We were like a team and this was a campaign. . . . I was the cause of all the trouble but I was also a member of the team. We were holding hands" (1985, p. 88). It should be evident that such involvement would encourage and empower patients toward self-care—which is, after all, authentic nursing care.

CONCLUSION

Nursing education prepares students for both taking care of patients and fostering their self-care. Taking care of patients, to be justified, must be given only when the patient is unable to care for him or herself. When patients are able to care for themselves and yet dependent care is given, care is taken *from* the patient. When nurses help patients learn self-care, they are practicing authentic care.

To enable nurses to give authentic care, nursing education needs to place greater stress on the humanities, which, in contrast to the stress on actuality in the sciences, focus on the possibilities of what could be and should be. Humanistic study also explores human experience, which should help nurses deal with the experience of illness in patients rather than reducing their experience and often themselves to a scientifically defined category of disease to be treated. Illness is experienced by patients as reducing their ability for self-care. By helping students encourage patients to see the possibilities for self-care, nursing faculty actually introduce humanistic understanding into actual nursing practice.

Helping patients to see the possibilities in their lived world requires that students develop personal relationships with patients and communicate openly with them concerning their experiences. For students to adequately explore possibilities for self-care with patients, they need time to get to know particular patients and to become comfortable in communicating with them concerning possibilities for a better life. Open communications enhance the opportunities for students to discuss with patients the meaning of their lives and their relationships with persons who make their lives meaningful. Such discussions empower students to give authentic care by helping patients discover possibilities for resuming that self-care which is essential to authentic human being.

REFERENCES

Benner, P., & Wrubel, J. (1989). *The primacy of caring.* Menlo Park, CA: Addison-Wesley.

Concept Media (Producer). (1989). *Hopelessness* [Filmstrip]. Irvine, CA: Concept Media.

Heidegger, M. (1972). *Being and time* (J. Macquarrie & E. Robinson, Trans.). New York: Harper & Row. (Original work published 1927).

Kesey, L. (1973). *One flew over the cuckoo's nest.* New York: Viking.

Orem, D. (1980). *Nursing: Concepts of practice* (2d ed.). New York: McGraw-Hill.

Ortega Y Gasset, J. (1960). *What is philosophy?* New York: Norton.

Rawlinson, M. C. (1982). Medicine's discourse and the practice of medicine. In V. Kestenbaum (Ed.), *The humanity of the ill* (pp. 69–85). Knoxville: University of Tennessee Press.

Scudder, J. R., Jr., & Bishop, A. H. (1986). The moral sense and health care. In A-T. Tymieniecka (Ed.), *Moral sense in the communal significance of life. Analecta Husserliana, 20* (pp. 125–158). Dordrecht-Boston: D. Reidel.

Zaner, R. (1985). How the hell did I get here?: Reflections on being a patient. In A. H. Bishop & J. R. Scudder, Jr. (Eds.), *Caring, curing, coping: Nurse, physician, patient relationships.* Tuscaloosa, AL: University of Alabama Press.

7

The Meaning of Human Care and the Experience of Caring in a University School of Nursing

Cathy Appleton

Education in the United States is the source of enormous debate and discussion. Dialogue about educational aims, standards, and practices has been revived because of a renewed interest in the merits of a liberal arts education. This renewed emphasis on the value of a liberal arts foundation as the preparation for professional nursing education challenges educators of nursing. Sakalys and Watson (1986) claimed the responsibility of a university school of nursing is to prepare the highest level of health professional who is well-educated, knowledgeable, and capable of making informed and wise human health care judgments.

Throughout history, professional nurses have spirited the cause of excellence in education, research, and practice. In keeping with nursing's tradition of excellence, Sigma Theta Tau (1987) addressed the issues paramount for nursing to enact a preferred future. Its recommendations focused on restructuring the profession to reflect nursing's value, mission, and contribution to the world community. The report specifically identified the importance of a new world view of nursing education, which must be constituted from a consideration of all persons involved in the process of education for professional nursing practice as well as the revision of current teaching methods. One position strongly endorsed was the preparation of professional nurses at an elevated level.

An informed perspective about the process of education and about the culture in which social behavior and intellectual activity ensue is necessary for restructuring academic communities. Transformation through evolution flourishes when educators are challenged to envision and espouse new philosophical perspectives, epistemologies, ontologies, and onticologies. The profession of nursing has a remarkable history of transforming persons, communities, organizations, and societies at large (Reverby, 1987). One of the most notable accomplishments was the creation of programs of study designed to formally educate students in the art and science of nursing at a time when formal education for women was generally denied. It was a time when the majority of what women learned was informally taught or occurred through instruction in the home (1987).

Recently, nurse scholars (Leininger, 1980; Gaut, 1983; Ray, 1981; Watson, 1979) have imagined a preferred future for nursing. They have heralded the science of nursing as one grounded in humanity. In keeping with this philosophical commitment, nursing's social mission of health promotion becomes possible only when the essence of nursing, which is caring, is recognized and expressed (Leininger, 1980; Ray, 1981; Watson, 1979). Caring, as the moral ideal of nursing, is nursing's unique contribution to humankind (Watson, 1985) and has the potential to transform health care. The challenge to create a new world view is based on recognizing the profession's contribution of human caring as unique to nursing (Roach, 1984).

An emphasis on excellence complemented with a new world view based on caring as the essence of nursing warrants novel and innovative inquiry into practice and education. Imaginative approaches to curriculum development will create opportunities to develop programs that educate prospective nurses whose practice will reflect the moral ideal, social mission, and essence of the profession. Noddings (1988) believed the moral orientation to teaching and the aim of education must be grounded in caring. She suggested that to approach education from a perspective of caring, teachers, teacher-educators, students, and researchers need time to engage in modeling, dialogue, practice, and confirmation (p. 229). Bevis (1989) believed caring must be present to create educational environments enabling self-actualization and fulfillment.

The manner of nurturing students and creating academic environments where caring is valued, experienced, and taught calls for an examination of the process and context in which human care knowledge is actualized. There is no research addressing the meaning and experience of caring in academic institutions that offer programs in nursing. The art and science of nursing could be advanced by research about the experience of caring during a professional education and within an academic setting. A critical look at how the ideal of caring is experienced in educational organizations has not been considered. Therefore, the goal of this research is to enhance knowledge about caring in an academic setting and to contribute to a new world view about nursing education based on a moral ideal of caring.

This study purports to describe the meaning of human care and the experience of caring from the perspective of doctoral students during their educational experience in a program of nursing. A qualitative research design using phenomenology was chosen and a purposive sample of two doctoral students from a National League of Nursing (NLN)-accredited program was selected. Data analyzed from the interviews uncovered themes of the meaning of human care and the lived experience of caring. As a result, the unity of the meaning of the lived experience of caring within the situation of doctoral nursing education was uncovered.

This study enhances understanding about phenomenology, presents a new world view about education, and conceptualizes academic organizations as cultures reflecting norms, traditions, and values that influence the experience of education. A synopsis of the philosophical foundation for phenomenology is introduced and a literature review describes a new world view about education. The concept of organizations as cultures is presented and substantiated as a metaphor useful to conceptualize how caring can transform educational institutions.

CONTEXT OF THE STUDY

Philosophical Foundation of the Research Methodology

Advancing nursing as a human science demands a new scientific approach that must address the study of human experience as it is lived (Ray, 1987). Qualitative methodology permits the researcher to address science from a human perspective and to discover what it means to be human by analyzing the descriptions of human experience. One qualitative method used to study the meaning of human experience (phenomena) is phenomenology.

Husserl first proposed this method as a creative attempt to apprehend meaning through studying human experience. He attempted to comprehend phenomena of living in a linguistic description that is holistic, analytic, precise, and universal (Ray, 1987, p. 169). An important distinction of phenomenology from other qualitative approaches is its philosophical basis, which originated with an existential phenomenological view emphasizing a person as unique, possessing potential, and experiencing opportunity for change. What is studied is phenomena as opposed to things in themselves (Oiler, 1986). The major difference between qualitative and quantitative methods is how the world of everyday lived experience is viewed. Qualitative research occurs within a natural context as compared with the contrived situations of quantitative methods (Cohen, 1987). Phenomenology is recognized as one of the most valuable approaches for uncovering meaning and describing experience.

Phenomenology strives to reveal the essence of understanding meaning in experience (Munhall, 1989). Phenomenological description is inherent on perspective given in experience and presented through description. Therefore, the interview technique was selected and the processes of structural reflection and description were used to discover the world as perceived by doctoral students. This process enabled the researcher to capture the phenomena of study and uncover the central themes of caring.

The Concept of Caring and Organizations as Cultures

Explicating the meaning of phenomena within a context is the purpose of qualitative research (Ray, 1989, p. 32). A consideration of the context is useful to further the discovery about what it means to be human. A concept such as culture enhances understanding about how organizations shape and are shaped by human experience (Thompson, 1967). Conceptualizing organizations as cultures is one way to contribute to knowledge development and further understanding about the meaning of being human.

Morgan (1986) claimed that the interactions of pluralities of persons in organizations contribute to the development of organizational cultures. He believed cultures have their own distinctive patterns reflecting norms, traditions, and values. How ideas, values, and symbols are related to and transform attitudes, feelings, and behavior is crucial to understanding culture and organizations as cultures (Ray, 1989, p. 32).

Caring is revealed in the beliefs, standards, and practices of an organization. The experience of caring elucidates the context in which it is lived. The phenomena of caring is one that can be studied from a phenomenological approach to person within the context of organizations as cultures.

Furthermore, health as purported by Parse (1981) suggests that the notion of health is one pertinent to understanding organizations as cultures. She defined health as a process of lived value priorities (1987, p. 159). Organizational health, including institutions of higher education and even academic disciplines, could be understood using a framework of organizations as cultures whose chosen value priorities are revealed as a way of living within that particular context. This approach offers possibilities for researching caring as a means of promoting organizational health.

Ray (1984), in keeping with a new world view, concluded that it is paramount for nursing to discover the meaning of care within specific cultural contexts of major social institutions. She believes a value of caring can transform organizations and revolutionize society at large (1981). Leininger (1986) specifically addressed the value of caring within the nursing profession. She claimed the concepts, principles, and practices related to human care have not been institutionalized as a normative expectation of nursing. Consequently, care cannot be ensured as a major aspect of nursing education and service.

Educational institutions conceived as organizational cultures can advance the aim of education in nursing and the moral orientation to teaching. Organizational culture reflects a shared meaning system (Ray, 1989). This meaning is conveyed and sustained within the organization. Ultimately, meaning contributes to and shapes perspectives about humanity and constructs knowledge integral for living in the world.

Cultures are always in transition and organizational cultures embody the changes in the values of the dominant culture (Ray, 1989, p. 33). If caring is a valued attribute for nurses, then its exemplification must be evident in educators of nursing (Rieman, 1987). Educators have the opportunity to enact these values and create academic cultures dominated by an ideal of caring. A critical examination of personal values is a way to initiate change and develop the ability for learning how to be humane (Carper, 1979).

The significance of understanding caring as an ideal way of being in the world and one that persons consciously strive to become is realized by studying caring as the essence of nursing. The metaphor of culture is useful for understanding organizations ontologically, specifically educational organizations where teaching and learning the art and science of nursing transpires. Caring offers hope for transforming nursing education and revolutionizing health care through restructuring the profession.

A New World View of Education in Nursing

Miller (1987) declared much of what is taught in higher education does not affect the deepest unconscious levels of the psyche, a process inherent in cognitive restructuring and moral development. To counteract such an experience, he believed that education must include a value for learning and restructuring. Miller maintained that a renewal process is necessary for personal, cognitive, scientific, and social advancement. He called for periodic reevaluation and reformulation of rules, traditions, beliefs, standards, and values guiding all manner of activity from social behavior to intellectual investigation as a means of renewal and ultimately advancement.

Miller's (1987) thesis about educational reform demonstrates the utility of thinking about organizations as cultures. Social context and cognition are significant aspects of education (1987) and culture (Morgan, 1986). The very basis of caring as a transformative force originates and develops within social context and cognition. The social context or caring ontology and the cognitive dimension or academic program in educational organizations must be addressed if caring is to be developed as both an ontology (social context) and epistemology (program).

Miller's notion of renewal is elaborated on by Campbell (cited in Flowers, 1988). Campbell suggested knowing begins with a journey inward. He believed a process of inner investigation is a universal phenomenon and one necessary for a holistic perspective. Inner investigation is necessary for restructuring to occur and requires an attitude that doubts what is real, and how one comes to know and be. Popper (1965) claimed this sort of inquiry contributes to the revision of existing knowledge and Kuhn (1970) believed it shaped scientific development.

The ideas of these scholars have had a tremendous influence on pedagogy and science. Their theories have contributed to the evolution of science and the exploration of human nature. Beliefs about perception, knowledge, and experience in the world have changed as a consequence of such scholarly contributions.

Restructuring education from this new world view challenges educators to consider the journey inward as a means to advance nursing education. An individual and collective journey inward can facilitate changes in educational aims, standards, and practice. Inquiry into novel ways of being can precipitate exploration of beliefs not formerly advanced in education. The process of actualizing knowledge, creating nurturing environments, and developing a context where learning is experienced through caring offers hope for advancing the discipline of nursing.

If it is the teacher's role to broaden, restructure, and transform a student's conceptual and normative frameworks (Popper, 1965), it is implicit that educators must initiate this process by first questioning what is and then what could be. Bevis (1989) believed caring must be present in the teacher-student relationship if the self-actualization process described by Popper is to occur. Mayeroff (1971) believed the primacy of caring is growth and self-actualization. An analysis of the literature on the philosophy of education reveals a common distinguishable theme of learning as growth and self-actualization. This same theme exists in the majority of the literature about caring (Ray, 1981).

The emphasis on growth and self-actualization as a dimension of learning and caring offers a new perspective on the experience of education and the context in which education transpires. Educational reform and organizational development rests on the value for learning based on an ethic of caring. This unique perspective can contribute to the restructuring of the profession through education in nursing.

RESEARCH APPROACH

Data Generation

This study focused on caring within an organizational culture of academia. The conceptual framework developed in this chapter was held in abeyance (bracketed) when data were generated from the interviews and initially analyzed for emerging themes and subthemes. The conceptual framework did provide a reference for understanding the goal, purpose, and groundwork for the research question, however. It also demonstrated the limited knowledge about the meaning of caring in an educational setting. These findings have the potential for contributing to a body of knowledge about caring in nursing education. The literature review was conducted after the data analysis and provided a confirmation for the unity of meaning uncovered.

A qualitative research design using phenomenology was selected as the most appropriate method to answer the research question. The phenomenological method delineated by Van Manen (1984) and described by Ray (1987) provided the guiding structure for analyzing the transcripts. Themes emerged and further reflection uncovered the essence of the lived experience.

The setting of the study was a NLN-accredited university school of nursing. Two doctoral students volunteered and consented to tape-recorded interviews to discuss the meaning of human care and the experience of caring from their perspectives as students. Both partici-pants agreed to attempt to capture moments of their experience of caring through the use of photography for another aspect of the study.

DATA ANALYSIS AND RESULTS

Data Generation

The two participants in the study were interviewed for 60 minutes. The interviews were open dialogues about the meaning of human care and the experience of caring during a program of education in nursing. The technique of talk-turning was used to elaborate on cues and ques-tion, in depth, the experience described during the interview process. Data from the interviews were transcribed and prepared for analysis by using a computer program (Seidel, Kjolseth, & Seymour, 1988).

Credibility of the study was assessed using qualitative guidelines for determining validity and reliability. The four criteria used were truth value, applicability, consistency, and neutrality suggested by Lincoln and Guba (1985). These criteria guided the researcher's activity during the conduct of the study. They stem from a naturalistic paradigm and are appropriate when evaluating the credibility of knowledge claims generated within a phenomenological paradigm of science.

Qualitative research methodologies are viewed within the context of the purpose of the research. Phenomenology as a qualitative methodol-ogy is used to uncover the meaning of human experience (Munhall, 1989). Since phenomenology accepts all experiences as valid sources of knowledge for the participants living the experience, each experience communicated to the researcher is valid (Ray, 1987). Therefore, quality of evidence refers to how well the study represented the lived reality as experienced by the participants.

Data Analysis

The specific methodological analyses used in this study were: cen-tering on the lived experience, holding in abeyance (bracketing) one's scientific presuppositions about the phenomenon, talking with the persons about the meaning of an experience, developing themes from investigating general essences from the recorded dialogues, and reflecting on the meaning of the whole as it is experienced. The recognition of patterns that unfolded from the particular facilitated the coming to know the whole of the meaning. The significance of the human experience was highlighted by using the language of the participants. The thematic analysis uncovered the themes that later provided the essence of the lived experience of caring. Deep reflection provided the opportunity to intuit about the universal meaning of being (Ray, 1987).

Development of Themes of Caring

Through the process of structured reflection on the students' descriptions of the meaning of human care and the experience of caring, characterizing themes about the expressions and process of caring unfolded. Tables 1 and 2 illustrate these central themes. The reported experiences of human caring in nursing education evolved into three significant aspects unified within the whole. Caring was expressive, a process, and had an environmental dimension. Expressions of caring for the other person involved treating him or her with respect, understanding his or her interdependence, helping him or her to grow, and letting him or her become. Caring was described as a process of commitment, involvement, and belonging. The experience of caring occurred within space, place, and time. Participants described the organizational structure and the notions of space, place, and time as the environmental dimension of the experience.

Deep structured reflection enabled the researcher to analyze the meaning of human care as a way of being concerned for treating the other person with respect for his or her individuality through understanding the other person's interdependence and helping the other to grow and letting the other person become. Although the unity of meaning of human care emphasized self-in-relation-to-other, the participants stated caring included self-care. Therefore, expressions of caring entailed expressions toward self and other.

Human care as a way of being concerned suggests an attitude of compassion is necessary for conveying the expression of caring. The caring expressions arise from a way of being concerned for self and others. Again, the way that caring is conveyed is through expressions arising from a compassionate attitude. This finding indicated that compassion is an ontology.

Table 1
Expressions of Caring

Themes	Theme Summary
Treating	Caring is treating the other person with respect for his or her individuality.
Understanding	Caring is understanding the other person's interdependence.
Helping	Caring is helping the other person to grow.
Letting	Caring is letting the other person become.

The process of caring emerged from the analysis of the descriptions about the experience and included commitment, involvement, and belonging for the purpose of becoming. Participants related that the process was a simultaneous one opposed to a linear sequential phenomenon. Subthemes surfacing from the rich descriptions further portrayed the essence of the process. The experience of caring lived by doctoral students of nursing was "sensing being in place and feeling belonging."

The process of caring depicted in Table 2 was intrinsic to a person's experience of becoming. A sense of being in place and feeling belonging was experienced as caring. Caring was known through sensing being in place and feeling belonging. When this happened, a perspective of growth of being, referred to as becoming, occurred. Ultimately the feeling of belonging (connected) facilitated a person's understanding of what it meant to be human. Knowledge of belonging gave meaning to what was taught and to the experience of learning. Apprehension of humanity of self is a form of aesthetic knowing (Carper, 1978) because it occurred when the student perceived, sensed, and felt connected to another. Therefore, caring as an epistemology is known aesthetically. Consequently, bringing forth the capacity (compassion) to express oneself-in-relation (caring) is a fundamental ontology and an epistemology, where the epistemology is inclusive of aesthetic knowing.

The meaning and experience of caring described by the participants emerged as a way of being in the world with other people. When caring is expressed, the experience enhances the other's becoming. A sense of being in place and feeling belonging occurs and this is how caring is known.

Table 2
The Process of Caring

Themes	Subthemes	Descriptions
Commitment	Potential	"I certainly sense in my colleagues at school, among students and faculty, the commitment toward putting forth the energy toward developing for each one of us our own potential."
	Reciprocal	"I think it's truly more reciprocal with both." "It's a two way kind of thing."
	Genuine	"I think there's genuine reciprocal caring among the students for each other."
Involvement	Personal	"I think we relate to the faculty here a lot on a real personal level and there's a real relationship there that's developed with the faculty."
	Spiritual	"Caring is something that's given more to the spiritual, holistic realm and you can pick up vibes from certain people."
	Holistic	"I feel ultimately more cared for, more holistically cared for by certain persons than others."
	Freedom	"Caring is the freedom to express ourselves and time to express ourselves rather than just having the faculty present and we sit back and absorb what is being said."
Belonging	Reassuring	"It's kind of reassuring."
	Comforting	"The feeling of being cared for, I think is comfort."
	Knowing	"I've just learned a tremendous amount with the whole process." "There's just some way we're on the same wave length and you know, so it happens."
	Connected	"The experience of caring is being in place and feeling connected."

Development of a Context of Caring

Data from the in-depth interviews revealed a distinct and yet integrally related meaning of caring within the context of the unity of the whole. Participants freely discussed caring as a personal, relational, situational, and environmental phenomenon encompassing caring for oneself (personal). Elaboration on the relational dimension of the experience included a variety of relationships within the educational experience. Participants discussed the relational aspects of the experience of caring in depth. These relationships occurred among students and among students and faculty. The nature of the relationships included person to person, person to group, and person to organization. Most descriptions focused on the person-to-person and person-to-group experience. They acknowledged a relationship between self and the organization that would be inclusive of aspects of the environment.

The situations identified involved such teaching-learning encounters as classroom experiences, advisory committee meetings, academic advisement, and scholarly forums. Organized social events and spontaneous socialization occasions also were referred to as situational.

The environmental phenomenon included the aspects of time, place, and space. The organizational bureaucracy was also considered an environmental phenomenon. Structural arrangements conducive to caring included decreasing the levels of complex hierarchy. A strong sense of ability to communicate and an identifiable purpose were essential ingredients in creating structural arrangements conducive for caring to occur. These findings suggest a need to design academic organizations to reflect a structure conducive for caring. Perhaps an ontology of compassion coupled with an ethic of caring will expose new organizational designs and modifications.

The desire for sufficient time to express and engage in a process of caring was essential. Adequate and pleasing surroundings were important when reflecting a caring environment. Designated places to socialize were extremely critical for feeling valued and recognized. Ultimately, these places contributed to feeling a sense of belonging.

The model in Figure 1 illuminates the context of caring as a whole. It illustrates the unity of the experience of the meaning of caring in education. Therefore, it is referred to as pedagogical caring.

Figure 1
Pedagogical Caring

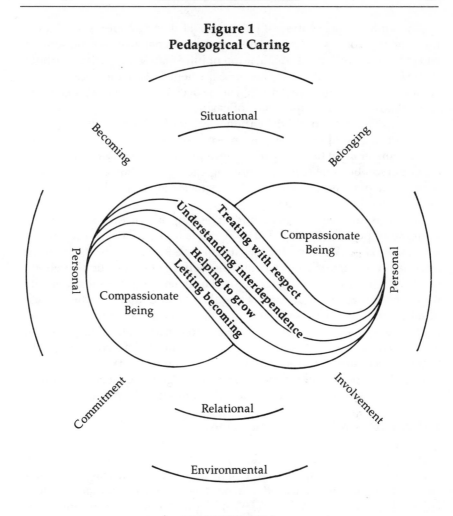

DISCUSSION

This study portrayed the magnitude of caring for the transformation of personal potential. Expressions of caring transpired within the personal, relational, situational, and environmental dimensions of being. The interconnectedness of these dimensions created and influenced a sense of belonging. Belonging gave meaning to the process of education and coming to know. Knowing one is cared for and about was essential for self-growth and stemmed from a feeling of belonging.

The students' perception of being cared for and about was critical to forming relations, situations, and an environment where self-creation and cultivation occurred. Acquisition of information may ensue without the experience of caring. However, experience of caring is tied to the student's becoming. Therefore, the process of becoming occurred through knowing the experience of caring.

The opportunity to discover the meaning of caring in nursing practice is contingent upon the experience of caring during a student's educational program. The ability to design a practice of nursing that lets the other person become through knowing caring is enhanced when a student has a professional educational experience from which to assign meaning and understanding.

Caring is an activity whose understanding is central to the understanding of person (Mayeroff, 1965) and is foundational to the profession of nursing (Watson, 1985). Curtin (1979) stated the purpose of nursing is not scientific but moral, "the welfare of other human beings" (p. 2). Noddings (1984) holds a similar belief about education. She professed the aim of education is moral and contended that the process of educating must be conducted in a thoroughly moral way. She purported caring was the approach needed to create a moral orientation. Therefore, education for nurses in preparation for a professional life requires recognition and acknowledgement of the significance of caring during this experience. Educators are challenged to conceive of opportunities to develop caring from the basic ontology of compassion.

Reformation in Nursing Education

New approaches and fresh ideas tempered with courage will illuminate and embellish this ontology. The participants in this study suggested caring is communicated in many ways, but that a person-oriented approach was critical. Buber's (1958) extrapolation of the notion of "I-thou" was congruent with the descriptions cited in this study. The roles of teacher and student dissipated when relations, situations, and the environment were created from a person-centered approach. Role emphasis and enactment could interfere with a person-centered approach, depending on the teachers' philosophy of education.

Pivotal to the caring relationship was the notion of freedom as the way of being involved with the other person. Caring was the freedom to be who one is, and education the means that augments becoming through a commitment to develop a person's potential for living a meaningful life. Noddings (1984) claimed that "the student is infinitely more important than the subject matter" (p. 176). She posited that teachers who are caring recognize that students will learn what they please. Although teachers can force students to respond in certain ways, eventually students will choose what is important to them for living their own lives. The outcome of this study supported Noddings's contention and demonstrated that caring enabled students to find meaning in the content selected for consideration in an academic program. Once meaning was found, then a value about the knowledge was created and insight into its importance for living was established.

Students reported teachers who expressed caring were willing to work with students by giving guidance and support to them. These teachers encouraged students to pursue their valued and unique interests. Furthermore, these teachers wanted students to do well and offered support through confirming the value each student contributed. Consequently, students felt free to engage these teachers in dialogue and critique of the students' ideas.

Teaching-learning encounters that enhanced the experience of caring entailed creating opportunities for students to meet their academic aspirations. Crucial for success was the time to understand and reflect during the teaching-learning experience. Opportunities for dialogue as opposed to complete lecture format were intrinsic to comprehending through exploration, freely sharing novel ideas, and freedom to express oneself. Participants reported smaller class sizes were critical to this process.

Faculty leadership to incarnate caring shaped and characterized the class. When faculty were caring, expectations were clearly communicated and criticism was constructive, contributing to a feeling of confirmation. Multiple opportunities to achieve academic aspirations existed.

These descriptions corroborated Noddings's (1984) thesis about commitment, cooperative engagement, dialogue, and confirmation. Moreover, they illuminate the interrelationship that exists in nursing education between freedom, possibility, and imagination. They highlight the relevance of Greene's (1988) argument that the creation of freedom must be achieved through continued resistance to the forces that limit, shape, and circumscribe oppression in our educational systems.

CONCLUSION

This study has described and analyzed the meaning and experience of caring during doctoral education in nursing. Fundamental expressions

of caring and a caring process were uncovered using the phenomenological method. Personal, relational, situational, and environmental dimensions revealed the nature of the context. A model of pedagogical caring
was developed to augment the understanding of caring as a whole.

Reformation in nursing education argued for a broadened perspective about the educational process and culture in which social behavior
and intellectual activity occur. Transformation of educational institutions and programs of nursing challenged administrators, educators,
and students to provide new ways of being, thinking, and experiencing.
An ontology of compassion was identified to be crucial for creating
caring relationships, situations, and academic environments.

Human care knowledge is advanced through nursing when caring is
experienced in academic life. The relevance of learning is realized in
knowing the value of knowledge for living a life of meaning. The quest
for excellence in the profession of nursing is contingent upon the education of future scholars, researchers, and practitioners. An ontology,
epistemology, and axiology of caring is no longer a mystery. It is merely
a matter of the challenge for the future.

REFERENCES

American Nurses' Association. (1975). *Human rights guidelines for nurses in clini-cal and other research.* Kansas City, MO: ANA.

Bevis, E. (1989). *Curriculum building in nursing.* New York: NLN Publications.

Buber, M. (1958). *I and thou.* New York: Scribners.

Carper, B. (1978). Fundamental patterns of knowing in nursing. *Advances in Nursing Science, 1*(1), 13–23.

Carper, B. (1979). The ethics of caring. *Advances in Nursing Science, 1*(2), 11–19.

Cohen, M. (1987). A historical overview of the phenomenologic movement. *Image, 19*(1), 31–34.

Curtin, L. (1979). The nurse as advocate: A philosophical foundation for nurs-ing. *Advances in Nursing Science, 1*(3), 1–10.

Flowers, B. (Ed.). (1988). *Joseph Campbell: The power of the myth.* New York: Doubleday.

Gaut, D. (1983). Development of a theoretically adequate description of caring. *Western Journal of Nursing Research, 5*(4), 313–324.

Greene, M. (1988). *The dialectic of freedom.* New York: Teachers College Press.

Kuhn, T. (1970). *The structure of scientific revolutions.* Chicago, IL: University of Chicago Press.

Leininger, M. M. (1980). Caring: A central focus of nursing and health care services. *Nursing and Health Care, 1*(1), 135–143.

Leininger, M. M. (1986). Care facilitation and resistance factors in the culture of nursing. *Topics in Clinical Nursing, 8*(2), 1–11.

Lincoln, Y., & Guba, E. (1985). *Naturalistic inquiry.* Beverly Hills, CA: Sage.

Mayeroff, M. (1965). On caring. *International Philosophy Quarterly, 5,* 462–474.

Mayeroff, M. (1971). *On caring.* New York: Harper & Row.

Miller, L. (1987). The other side of learning. *Thought and Action: The National Education Association Higher Education Journal, 3*(1), 87–96.

Morgan, G. (1986). *Images of organization.* Beverly Hills, CA: Sage.

Munhall, P. (1989). Philosophical ponderings on qualitative research methods in nursing. *Nursing Science Quarterly, 2*(1), 20–28.

Noddings, N. (1984). *Caring: A feminine approach to ethics and moral education.* Berkeley: University of California Press.

Noddings, N. (1988). An ethic of caring and its implications for instructional arrangements. *American Journal of Education, 97*(2), 215–229.

Oiler, C. (1986). Phenomenology: The method. In P. L. Munhall & C. J. Oiler (Eds.)., *Nursing research: A qualitative perspective* (pp. 69–84). Norwalk, CT: Appleton-Century-Crofts.

Parse, R. (1981). *Man-living-health: A theory of nursing.* New York: Wiley.

Parse, R. (1987). Man-living-health. In R. R. Parse (Ed.), *Nursing science: Major paradigms, theories and critiques* (pp. 159–180). Philadelphia: Saunders.

Popper, K. (1965). *Conjectures and refutations: The growth of scientific knowledge.* New York: Basic Books.

Ray, M. (1981). A philosophical analysis of caring within nursing. In M. M. Leininger (Ed.), *Caring: An essential human need* (pp. 25–36). Thorofare, NJ: Slack.

Ray, M. (1987). Technological caring: A model in critical care. *Dimensions of Critical Care Nursing, 6*(3), 166–173.

Ray, M. (1989). The theory of bureaucratic caring for nursing practice in the organizational culture. *Nursing Administration Quarterly, 13*(2), 31–42.

Rieman, D. (1987). The essential structure of a caring interaction: Doing phenomenology. In P. L. Munhall & C. J. Oiler (Eds.), *Nursing research: A qualitative perspective* (pp. 85–108). Norwalk, CT: Appleton-Century-Crofts.

Reverby, S. (1987). *Ordered to care: The dilemma of American nursing.* Cambridge: Cambridge University Press.

Roach, Sr., S. (1984). *Caring: The human mode of being. Implications for nursing* (Perspectives in Caring Monograph No. 1). Toronto: University of Toronto, Faculty of Nursing.

Sakalys, J., & Watson, J. (1986). Professional education: Post-baccalaureate education for professional nursing. *Journal of Professional Nursing, 2*(2), 91–97.

Seidel, J., Kjolseth, R., & Seymour, E. (1988). *The ethnograph: A program for the computer-assisted analysis of test-based data* [Computer program]. Littleton, CO: Qualis Research Associates (Version 3.0).

Sigma Theta Tau International. (1987). *Arista: Direction for action looking toward 2010*, pp. 16–21.

Thompson, J. (1967). *Organizations in action.* New York: McGraw-Hill.

Watson, J. (1979). *Nursing: The philosophy and science of caring.* Boston: Little, Brown.

Watson, J. (1985). *Nursing: Human science and human care. A theory of nursing.* Norwalk, CN: Appleton-Century-Crofts.

8

The Essential Structure of a Caring and an Uncaring Encounter with a Teacher: The Perspective of the Nursing Student

Sigrídur Halldórsdóttir

Love:
The professional's perspective.

Love is gentle
kind
and
knowledgeable.

Love is sharing
hoping
and
caring.

Love is fair
joyful
and
eternal.

Sigrídur Halldórsdóttir
February 8, 1989

Historical belief in nursing as a caring profession and traditional values of caring and compassion embodied in the word "nursing" are worth preserving for future generations of nurses and patients (Beyers, 1987; Sample, 1987). An awareness of and sensitivity to caring and uncaring backed by systematic investigation of these phenomena in nursing care and nursing education offer one of the greatest hopes for improving health care services and for advancing the discipline of nursing (Halldórsdóttir, 1988; Leininger, 1984).

It has been suggested that care is the essence and the central, unifying, and dominant domain that characterizes nursing (Leininger, 1984). Caring has been seen as a nursing term, representing all the facets used to deliver nursing care to clients (Eriksson, 1987; Watson, 1985). It has even been suggested that caring means the same as *nursing*, which is derived from "to nourish" (Griffin, 1983). However, nurses have expressed concern over how increasingly difficult it is for nursing to sustain its caring ideology (Dossey, 1982; Fry, 1988; Kelly, 1988; Miller, 1987; Moccia, 1988; Ray, 1981). Yet, given our space-age technology, the need for caring in nursing today is paramount (Benner & Wrubel, 1989; Carper, 1979; Henderson, 1985; Kelly, 1984).

The importance of offering nursing students opportunities to enhance their caring has been suggested in nursing literature (Astill-McNish, 1984; Stein, 1986). It has even been proposed that the primary aim of every educational institution and effort must be the maintenance and enhancement of caring (Noddings, 1984). Nursing education literature has, however, dealt minimally with the caring imperative in education. If nursing teachers want to be advocates and models of caring and if they want to understand the role of human caring in the teaching-learning process, they must become knowledgeable about caring and uncaring from the student's point of view.

This study purported to explore the phenomena of caring and uncaring in nursing education, as perceived by former students, so as to know and understand these phenomena more fully. The research question for the study was: What is the essential structure of a caring and an uncaring encounter with a teacher, from the perspective of the recipient of nursing education?

The underlying perspective for the study was symbolic interactionism. Herbert Blumer (1969), a leading exponent of this theory, defines symbolic interaction as that which occurs between human beings who interpret or define each other's actions instead of just reacting to them. Their responses are based on the meanings they attach to such actions (Riehl, 1980; Lindesmith, Strauss, & Denzin, 1978).

METHODOLOGY

The phenomenological perspective of qualitative research theory guided the methodological approach to the study, in which theoretical sampling, intensive unstructured interviews, and constant comparative analysis were used. Nine former nursing students participated in the study, and since the BSN degree is an entry to practice in Iceland, all have a university education. Four have a BSN degree, four have a MSN degree, and one is working toward a PhD. Data were collected through 16 in-depth, open-ended interviews that were tape-recorded and transcribed verbatim for each participant. The researcher saw the participants in the study as co-researchers and through intersubjective interaction, or true dialogue, the essential description of a caring and an uncaring encounter was constructed (Halldórsdóttir, 1989).

THE ESSENTIAL STRUCTURE OF A *CARING* STUDENT-TEACHER ENCOUNTER

The essential structure of a caring encounter with a teacher from the nursing student's perspective has four basic components: the teacher's professional caring approach; the resulting mutual trust and professional teacher-student working relationship; and finally, the positive student responses to the caring encounter (see Figure 1).

Professional Caring Teacher Approach

From the co-researchers' perspective, the caring teacher is professionally competent, has genuine concern for the student as a studying person, has a positive personality, and is professionally committed. These essential elements are perceived by the co-researchers as evidence of professional caring.

Professional Competence. The co-researchers emphasized that professional competence was an essential component of professional caring. They indicated that caring without competence was of little value to them as students. Professional competence essentially includes professional knowledge and experience, professional presentation of content, high standards for self and students, and academic fairness. Many co-researchers emphasized that competence alone often has limited value. In fact, they argued that a teacher has to be both competent and

Figure 1
The Essential Structure of a Caring Student-Teacher Encounter:
The Nursing Student's Perspective

Teacher's Approach	Trust	Relationship Formation	Student Responses
Teacher's professional caring: ⇒	Mutual trust ⇒	Developing teacher-student working relationship while keeping a respectful distance: ⇒	Positive responses to professional caring
Professional competence		*Developing a relationship:*	Sense of acceptance and self-worth
Genuine concern		–Initiating attachment	
Positive personality		–Mutual acknowledgment	Personal and professional growth and motivation
Professional commitment		of personhood	
		–Professional intimacy	
		–Negotiation of learning	Appreciation and role-modeling
		outcomes	
		–Student goal-directed work	Long-term gratitude and respect
		–Graduation/separation	
		Keeping a respectful distance	

caring to be truly professional. Thus compassion is perceived as the kind of attitude necessary for true professional competence. This attitude or feeling is perceived as genuine concern for the student as a studying person.

Genuine Concern for the Student as a Studying Person. The co-researchers explicitly emphasized that genuine concern for the student was one of the most important aspects of true professional caring. It includes genuine respect for students, concern that they really learn, faith in students as studying persons, and, therefore, academic freedom. The teacher's genuine concern also includes being attentive to the individual student, giving professional confrontation or honest feedback, and being interested in the student's future.

Positive Personality. Related to genuine concern is the caring teacher's positive personality. The co-researchers' unanimously perceived that positive personality is an element of professional caring which is extremely important for an experience of a caring encounter with a teacher. The main positive personal characteristics described were *personal integrity*—being honest and genuine; *sharing and giving of self; attentiveness*—being totally involved and really listening; *flexibility;* and *humor.* The accounts clearly illustrate the co-researchers' perceptions of the importance of these positive personality traits. It seems to be important for students to have as their teachers positive and generous individuals.

Professional Commitment.   The last theme is the importance of the teacher's professional commitment. This important quality of professional caring is evidenced by the teacher's enthusiasm for own subject, sense of vision, high regard for nurses and nursing, professional activity, and search for excellence.

Mutual Trust

It was the co-researchers' perception that caring teachers trust their students, and that encountering a truly caring teacher created in them a sense of trust. This mutual trust is a necessary foundation for a professional teacher-student working relationship. For many co-researchers, this connection or development of a relationship was the fundamental difference between caring and uncaring.

Working Relationship

Developing a professional teacher-student working relationship while keeping a respectful distance involves two interrelated processes: developing a professional working relationship and keeping a respectful distance.

Development of a *professional teacher-student working relationship* can be conceptualized as a process involving six phases.

1. Initiating attachment requires effective communication and reaching out. If there is a lack of reciprocity in this phase, the attachment does not develop any further. Successful completion of this phase, however, means that both student and teacher are willing to enter a working relationship and the attachment development progresses toward the second phase.
2. Mutual acknowledgment of personhood means that both teacher and student remove the masks of anonymity and recognize each other as persons. This phase involves some mutual self-disclosure,

but only enough to personalize the encounter. It also involves mutual communication of acceptance, as well as mutual acknowledgment of each other's uniqueness as persons. Successful completion of this phase establishes the bond between the teacher and the student.

3. After acknowledging attachment, teacher and student develop boundaries in the working relationship, and the attachment progresses to a deeper level of professional intimacy, where the student feels safe enough to open up and speak the truth to the teacher—to share some of his or her explanatory model. It also means that the student feels free to ask the teacher questions concerning his or her present learning situation and trusts the teacher to be truthful in giving honest feedback. What makes this intimacy professional is the emphasis on keeping it to the educational domain. Only when professional intimacy has been developed is there a foundation for true negotiation of learning outcomes.

4. Negotiation of learning outcomes involves three steps: dialoguing, negotiating, and concluding. Negotiating learning outcomes means that the teacher appreciates the student as an independent individual. Treating the student as an equal is the foundation of dialoguing and negotiating, and gives the student the feeling that the teacher is on his or her side. One important task in negotiation, however, is that the teacher is supportive without nurturing too much dependence. Successful completion of this phase results in the student's own goal-directed work.

5. As a result of professional intimacy the teacher is better able to understand the student and his or her world. This understanding enables the teacher to work with the student as an equal toward their common goal, the student's learning. If the student does become dependent, the teacher fosters independence as soon as possible, to the point where the student no longer needs the teacher. This implies that the goal of the professional teacher-student working relationship is that the student becomes able enough to stop being a student, that the student graduates.

6. When the student graduates the professional teacher-student working relationship is terminated. The working relationship is often quite strong at that point. In fact, sometimes the caring teacher invites the graduate to a new kind of relationship, which is closer to friendship, but is still situated within the academic world.

From the co-researchers' perspective, respectful distance is one of the main differences between personal and professional relationships. The co-researchers not only articulated their own need for professional distance, but also why they thought it was important for the teacher as well. They indicated that a professional working relationship serves a particular purpose in a particular setting or culture for a limited time, and attachment without respectful distance would therefore be inappropriate. They also seemed to consider the right amount of respectful distance an important part of professionalism. Consequently, developing a relationship without keeping a respectful distance was identified as lack of professionalism, and an evidence of caring that was not professional.

Positive Student Responses to Professional Caring

The co-researchers' responses to professional caring were many-sided. Four major themes were identified in their accounts.

Sense of Acceptance and Self-Worth.   Professional caring seems to give students a feeling of acceptance, and that they have worth in their own right. The professional teacher gets to know the student as a unique individual, not as a stereotype, and treats the student accordingly. Consequently, the student feels accepted, develops a positive self-image, and a sense of security. Furthermore, the caring teacher seems to be able to give students hope and optimism that encourages and challenges them to do better. The feeling of being cared for strengthens students and gives them more confidence.

Personal and Professional Growth and Motivation.   The caring teacher seems to motivate the student in an important way to learn and grow, both personally and professionally. The student develops increased interest in the subject and learns and grows, which gives him or her a sense of accomplishment and pride, a sense of achievement. The co-researchers' accounts illustrate how caring influences the student's ability to learn: both as a result of the teacher's encouragement and support, and because the student does not have to deal with negative emotions. Some co-researchers articulated the relief that they sensed when they felt cared for, and how being cared for diminished anxiety and gave them positive energy, motivating them to concentrate on learning.

Appreciation and Role-Modeling.   The co-researchers emphasized how much they appreciated the caring teacher. Professional caring not only results in a deep appreciation but also gives students a desire to model themselves on the caring teacher. Students seem to internalize the teacher's values and outlook, in a considerable way, which often results in a positive image of nursing and self as a nurse.

Long-Term Gratitude and Respect.   The co-researchers unanimously expressed sincere feelings of respect and gratitude toward the caring teacher. Even many years after the caring encounter, they still had that warm, positive feeling of respect and gratitude. It is clear from the co-researchers' accounts that the caring teacher was, and still is, a very special person in their minds.

THE ESSENTIAL STRUCTURE OF AN *UNCARING* STUDENT-TEACHER ENCOUNTER

The essential structure of an uncaring encounter with a teacher from the student's perspective has four basic components: the teacher's lack of professional caring; the resulting lack of trust; teacher-student detachment; and negative student responses to the uncaring encounter (see Figure 2).

Lack of Professional Caring

Perceived teacher indifference to the student as a studying person is defined as uncaring by the co-researchers. Four dimensions of an uncaring teacher approach were identified in the data, characterized by increased indifference, inattentiveness, and insensitivity to the student and his needs.

Lack of Professional Competence.   A teacher's lack of professional competence is perceived by the student as uncaring. From the co-researchers' perspective, lack of professional competence includes lack of professional knowledge and experience, lack of professional presentation, lack of commitment, lack of professional standards, and lack of respect for self and nursing. If the teacher also has some personal problems, this lack of professional competence becomes more prominent and disturbing for the student.

Lack of Concern.   When the teacher is unconcerned and insensitive to the students and their needs, the teacher is perceived by the student as inattentive and lacking in genuine concern. This attitude is characterized by lack of willingness to know the student, lack of interest in

Figure 2
The Essential Structure of an Uncaring Student-Teacher Encounter:
The Nursing Student's Perspective

Teacher's Approach	Trust	Relationship Formation	Student Responses
Teacher's lack of professional caring: ⇒	**Lack of trust** ⇒	**Teacher-student detachment with total distance** ⇒	**Negative responses to lack of professional caring:**
Lack of professional competence			*General reactions:*
Lack of concern			–Affective reactions
Demand for control and power			–Student coping strategies
Destructive behavior			–Long-term negative feelings and memories
			Specific reactions

teaching students, lack of willingness to acknowledge individual differences, and lack of respect for students.

Demand for Control and Power.   When the student senses a demand for control and power in the teacher, the teacher's indifference to the student as a studying person starts to become seriously disruptive for the student. The student experiences the teacher as a manipulative, inflexible, and authoritarian person, who sometimes even uses academic coercion. There is a lack of humanness in the teacher's approach to the student, and the student perceives the teacher as someone cold and unkind, as a conductor or overlord, rather than facilitator or catalyst. Demand for control and power involves a considerable negative feedback to the student. The most severe form of indifference, however, is a teacher's destructive behavior, where the social contact becomes severely destructive for the student.

Destructive Behavior.   This most severe form of indifference to the student as a studying person is characterized by various forms of unethical and inhumane attitudes, such as severe manipulation, showing contempt, and complete disrespect for the student. Being totally ignored as a person, being mistreated, ridiculed, and treated as a pest, constitutes a strong negative feedback for the student and involves a transference of considerable negative energy. The student feels that the teacher is against him or her, suffers, and feels victimized.

Lack of Trust

The perceived teacher indifference to the student as a studying person results in a lack of trust by the student, and there is no attachment formed between them. The result is a teacher-student detachment with total distance.

Detachment with Total Distance

The perceived indifference and lack of concern by the teacher makes the student distrustful, which leads to mutual avoidance. There is minimum verbal communication between the teacher and the student, and the nonverbal feedback is mostly negative.

Student Responses to Lack of Professional Caring

The co-researchers felt that uncaring encounters with teachers were discouraging and distressing experiences for them as students. Their responses were many-sided. Two major categories were identified in their accounts.

General Reactions.   The student's general *affective reactions* are diverse. At first the student is hoping for the best. It is apparent from the co-researchers' accounts that they expected their teachers to be caring. When they encountered uncaring teachers, therefore, their initial reactions were puzzlement and disbelief. Following the realization that they are indeed experiencing uncaring, the students seem to go through a stage of resentment and anger, and most often lose respect for the teacher.

Students have some *coping strategies and resources,* however. These include their own personal strength, supportive family and friends, fellow classmates, and the caring teachers. Thoughts about quitting, leaving the course, or leaving nursing altogether seem to be more frequent than thoughts about complaining. It is apparent that while still in the midst of the uncaring experience the student often fears retaliation for complaining. Complaining might even make the situation worse! By the time something is done about the complaint they will probably already have graduated anyway, seems to be the thought. However, some individual students or whole groups of students were brave enough to complain. Yet, in spite of many coping strategies and resources, the co-researchers still had some *negative feelings and memories* about the uncaring encounter. Although most co-researchers had tried to forgive the uncaring teacher, some admitted that they were probably more forgetful than forgiving.

Specific Reactions. Specific student reactions depend on the nature and degree of uncaring experienced. Reactions to *lack of professional competence* are mainly feelings of wasted time and energy; feeling ashamed belonging to, or in the process of belonging to, a profession that offers such teachers; and finally, some sense of pity. Reactions to *teacher's lack of concern* is mainly discouragement and uneasiness. Student reactions to *demand for control and power* are senses of being manipulated and feelings of vulnerability. Reactions to *teacher's destructive behavior* include uneasiness and fear, negative self-image, and, finally, despair and helplessness.

CONCLUSION

This study explored the essential structure of caring and uncaring encounters with teachers from the nursing student's perspective. Although "care" and "caring" have been used in the nursing literature for more than a century, only recently have nurses undertaken systematic philosophic and scientific investigation into these constructs (Ray, 1984). However, considerable evidence documents how influential caring and uncaring can be for the recipient, be it a patient or a student (Drew, 1986; Gadow, 1980, 1985; Gaut, 1983; Halldórsdóttir, 1988; Pauley, 1985; Pellegrino, 1985; Riemen, 1986a, 1986b; Rogers, 1969; Sarason, 1985; Siegel, 1986). At the same time, limited research is available on nursing students' experience of caring and uncaring during their nursing educations. Such studies could offer us hope for increased caring and decreased uncaring in these future care providers' learning experiences.

As one co-researcher stated:

> I think what people need most of all is a feeling of freedom, a true academic freedom, where you can grow, really grow, and become the person you best can be. But to allow that freedom the teacher has to be very professionally competent, really knowing what she or he is doing, and also having some faith in the individual. The attitude is that "a flower grows best if allowed free space to grow in, along with some warmth and nourishment." I think the human spirit is in a

way like a flower, but the uncaring teachers don't care for flowers, and some of them obviously hate human flowers.

> *Love must not be a matter of words or talk;*
> *it must be genuine,*
> *and show itself in action.*
>
> *I John 3:18*

REFERENCES

Astill-McNish, S. (1984). A sensitization program for geriatric nurses: Games that make you care. *The Canadian Nurse, 80*(3), 19–24.

Benner, P. & Wrubel, J. (1989). *The primacy of caring: Stress and coping in health and illness.* Menlo Park, CA: Addison-Wesley.

Beyers, M. (1987). Future of nursing care delivery. *Nursing Administrative Quarterly, 11*(2), 71–80.

Blumer, H. (1969). *Symbolic interactionism: Perspective and method.* Englewood Cliffs, NJ: Prentice-Hall.

Carper, B. (1979). The ethics of caring. *Advances in Nursing Science, 1*(3), 11–19.

Dossey, L. (1982). Consciousness and caring: Retrospective 2000. *Topics in Clinical Nursing, 3*(4), 75–83.

Drew, N. (1986). Exclusion and confirmation: A phenomenology of patients' experiences with caregivers. *IMAGE: Journal of Nursing Scholarship, 18*(2), 39–43.

Eriksson, K. (1987a). *Vårdandets idé.* Stockholm: Almqvist & Wiksell.

Eriksson, K. (1987b). *Pausen.* Stockholm: Almqvist & Wiksell.

Fry, S. (1988). The ethic of caring: Can it survive in nursing? *Nursing Outlook, 36*(1), 48.

Gadow, S. (1980). Existential advocacy: Philosophical foundation of nursing. In S. F. Spicker & S. Gadow (Eds.), *Nursing: Images and ideals.* New York: Springer-Verlag.

Gadow, S. (1985). Nurse and patient: The caring relationship. In A. H. Bishop & J. R. Scudder, Jr., *Caring, curing, coping: Nurse, physician, patient relationships.* Tuscaloosa, AL: University of Alabama Press.

Gaut, D. A. (1983). Development of a theoretically adequate description of caring. *Western Journal of Nursing Research, 5*(4), 313–324.

Griffin, A. P. (1983). A philosophical analysis of caring in nursing. *Journal of Advanced Nursing, 8*, 289–294.

Halldórsdóttir, S. (1988). *Caring and uncaring encounters in nursing practice: The patient's perspective.* Unpublished manuscript.

Halldórsdóttir, S. (1989). *Caring and uncaring encounters in nursing education: The student's perspective.* Unpublished manuscript.

Henderson, V. (1985). The essence of nursing in high technology. *Nursing Administration Quarterly, 9*(4), 1–9.

Kelly, L. S. (1984). High tech/touch—now more than ever. *Nursing Outlook, 32*(1), 15.

Kelly, L. S. (1988). The ethic of caring: Has it been discarded? *Nursing Outlook, 36*(1), 17.

Leininger, M. M. (1979). Foreword. In J. Watson, *Nursing: The philosophy and science of caring.* Boston: Little, Brown.

Leininger, M. M. (1981). *Caring: An essential human need.* Thorofare, NY: Slack.

Leininger, M. M. (1984). *Care: The essence of nursing and health.* Thorofare, NJ: Slack.

Lindesmith, A. R., Strauss, A. L., & Denzin, N. K. (1977). *Social psychology* (5th ed.). New York: Holt, Rinehart & Winston.

Miller, K. L. (1987). The human care perspective in nursing administration. *Journal of Nursing Administration, 17*(2), 10–12.

Moccia, P. (1988). At the faultline: Social activism and caring. *Nursing Outlook, 36*(1), 30–33.

Noddings, N. (1984). *Caring: A feminine approach to ethics & moral education.* Berkeley: University of California Press.

Pauley, C. (1985). Mask matter: How nurses' attitudes helped—and hurt—my recovery. *Journal of Christian Nursing, 5*(4), 25–26.

Pellegrino, D. D. (1985). The caring ethic: The relation of physician to patient. In A. H. Bishop & J. R. Scudder, Jr. (Eds.), *Caring, curing, coping: Nurse, physician, patient relationships.* Tuscaloosa, AL: University of Alabama Press.

Ray, M. (1981). A philosophical analysis of caring within nursing. In M. M. Leininger (Ed.), *Caring: An essential human need.* Thorofare, NJ: Slack.

Riehl, J. P. (1980). The Riehl interaction model. In J. P. Riehl & C. Roy (Eds.), *Conceptual models for nursing practice* (2d ed.). New York: Appleton-Century-Crofts.

Riemen, D. J. (1986a). Noncaring and caring in the clinical setting: Patients' descriptions. *Topics in Clinical Nursing, 8*(2), 30–36.

Riemen, D. J. (1986b). The essential structure of a caring interaction: Doing phenomenology. In P. L. Munhall & C. Oiler (Eds.), *Nursing research: A qualitative perspective.* Norwalk, CT: Appleton-Century-Crofts.

Rogers, C. R. (1969). *Freedom to learn.* Columbus, OH: Merrill.

Sample, S. A. (1987). Believe and achieve: The standard shall be excellence. *Nursing Administration Quarterly, 11*(2), 17–19.

Sarason, S. B. (1985). *Caring and compassion in clinical practice.* San Francisco: Jossey-Bass.

Siegel, B. S. (1986). *Love, medicine & miracles: Lessons learned about self-healing from a surgeon's experience with exceptional patients.* New York: Harper & Row.

Stein, A. P. (1986). Teaching nurses to care. *Nurse Educator, 11*(6), 4.

Watson, J. (1979). *Nursing: The philosophy and science of caring.* Boston: Little, Brown.

Watson, J. (1985). *Nursing: Human science and human care.* Norwalk, CT: Appleton-Century-Crofts.

9

Caring in Nursing Education: A Theoretical Blueprint

Mary Lou Sheston

Caring is a unifying focus for the study of nursing as a human science. Caring provides us with a new and different ontology for nursing and for society, an evolutionary perspective for developing new ways and patterns of knowing in the discipline (Moccia, 1988; Watson, 1987).

A body of knowledge about caring in nursing education is being developed in many exciting and diverse ways. New directions are being called for, and new models are evolving. We are changing our perceptions of what learning is, and are moving toward a greater concern with the process of education and the interpersonal relationships between teachers and students (Bevis, 1988; Moccia, 1988a). This chapter describes the development of a caring model for nursing education and the beginning investigation of auxiliary theory in support of the model.

MODEL DEVELOPMENT

Metatheoretical Perspectives

The development of a body of knowledge is an orderly, systematic process that progresses over time. Jerome Hage (1972) and Margaret

Newman (1979) clarify the process, providing a useful framework for theory building.

Hage (1972) delineates six critical elements of a theory and the contributions that each element makes toward theory development. Concepts, the building blocks of theory, describe and classify aspects of the phenomena of interest. Theoretical statements connect the concepts and assert relationships. This introduces the possibility of analysis. It is then necessary to provide clear definitions for the concepts. Theoretical definitions provide meaning for the concepts, and permit linkages to other theoretical ideas. Operational definitions provide for the observation of phenomena by specifying empirical indicators. These definitions establish reference points for "locating the concept."

Next, a clear rational for stated conceptual relationships needs to be developed. Hage (1972) calls this element "linkages," providing the why and the how for asserting particular relationships. This critical stage of theory development contributes plausibility and testability to the theory (p. 132).

As the theory develops, concepts and theoretical statements multiply, and the process of conceptual ordering is required. This final element provides for the elimination of tautology and inconsistency by pointing up any existing overlap between concepts, definitions, and relationship statements. The process is evolutionary developing in complexity and organization over time. A critical and creative dialectic between the theory elements results in the ongoing transformation of each.

Margaret Newman (1979) provides similar understanding of the knowledge-building process. The formulation of a conceptual model presents a matrix of abstract concepts and an organized way of looking at phenomena. The model suggests the kinds of questions to be asked and the relationships to be studied. A framework for theory development emerges. Direction is provided for the explication and identification of concepts and subconcepts relative to the phenomena of interest. Newman suggests that concepts and subconcepts be structurally grouped by specific characteristics into theoretical constructs. Constructs incorporate the meaning of concepts and provide variables that can be theoretically and operationally defined. Relationships between the variables are then proposed and investigated, and theoretical support for the model begins.

Newman (1979) reiterates that a model describes relationships in abstract conceptual ways; it is not testable. Its validity rests primarily on its usefulness in developing theory. It is necessary to describe auxiliary theory composed of carefully composed constructs. As in the evolutionary process described by Hage (1972), new sets of related concepts emerge, and new relationships are derived and tested.

Overview of a Caring Model

Initial development of a model of caring for nursing education provided a matrix of related concepts and relationships through the process of literature analysis and synthesis (Sheston, 1988a, 1988b). Caring in nursing education is conceptualized as an evolutionary, interpersonal process between a nurse educator (NE) and a nurse student (NS). The process incorporates experiences of caring interactions and transactions in a shared existential, phenomenological field called nursing education (Rogers, 1969; Watson, 1979). Both the NE and the NS become more, in a process of mutual evolution, change, and growth. This process or movement toward an ever-increasing human caring potential is conceptualized as transformation. The NE and the NS come to an expanded knowledge of self as caring beings; the educational process affirms and encourages the humanity of all involved (Buber, 1958; Moccia, 1988a; Putt, 1978; Watson, 1985).

Literature Support

An exploration of selected literature from philosophy, the behavioral sciences, and nursing provided indicators and concepts of caring for review, analysis, and synthesis. The language of the model was refined and clarified as concepts were grouped and structured and a gestalt of interrelationships was developed. This clustering activity allows for the organization of concepts into sets of variables or theoretical blocks, showing how the concepts may be interrelated (Blalock, 1969).

Humanistic and Existential Support. The works of Barrett (1962), Jones (1941), and Mead (1934) view the development of man's conscious sense of self as the most important aspect of his efforts to interact and identify with another. A conscious interactive process binds all humans in their social world of behaviors and experiences. Martin Buber (1958) and Gabriel Marcel (1971) provide support for existential approaches to meaningful interactions in the educational setting. Concepts of confirmation, love, and presence emerge. Buber sees mutual confirmation as the most important aspect of human growth. An I-thou relationship involves real knowledge of another, and requires openness, participation, and empathy. Like Buber, Marcel (1971) sees human interaction as being and doing with another, characterized by a sense of presence and availability. Fromm (1962) expands the idea of human confirmation to include elements of care, responsibility, and respect. Mayeroff (1971) views caring as a mutual human activity that involves helping another grow and actualize himself.

Education as a facilitative, growth-producing process is described clearly in the works of Carl Rogers (1951, 1957, 1961, 1965, 1969). Humanistic learning must include conditions of realness or genuineness, the presence of unconditional positive regard, and the quality of empathic understanding. Teachers are seen as catalysts in releasing the human capacities of both the educator and the student. Rogers (1975) calls caring or "prizing" a critical attitude for providing a climate that nurtures creativity and growth.

Carkhuff (1969) provides further development of Rogers's theory and describes a helping (caring) process as including facilitative conditions of understanding and action. Mutual growth depends on mutually perceived expectations and self-exploration. These writings lend support to a model of caring for nursing education that proposes a learning climate oriented to change and growth through a caring interpersonal process.

Support from Nursing Theory.   The works of Peplau (1952), Travelbee (1971), and Wiedenbach (1964) describe nursing as an interpersonal, helping process between a nurse and a patient. Travelbee theorized nursing as communication that establishes significant and meaningful experiences, including transcendence, empathy, sympathy and rapport.

The humanistic nursing theory of Paterson and Zderad (1988) proposes that nursing is a lived dialogue—an intersubjective transaction between a nurse and another. The art of nursing is characterized by synchronicity, intimacy, and mutuality, occurring in a time frame of here and now. These theorists, drawing from the work of Martin Buber (1958), describe characteristics of I-thou relating as including the offering of authentic presence, empathy, and mutual growth. Meaning depends on the mutual unfolding that develops from mutual interaction.

Leininger (1977, 1978) has developed a theory of nursing from her extensive anthropologic research. Nursing is viewed from a caring, transcultural perspective. Caring behaviors must be studied as the essential theoretical framework for practice. Leininger has developed a taxonomy of caring constructs that includes concepts of presence, trust, concern, interest, empathy, and enabling, facilitating behaviors.

Watson (1979) proposes a science of caring in nursing as an interpersonal human activity. She identifies ten factors as a structure for studying and understanding caring. They include the formulation of a humanistic-altruistic system of values; the instillation of faith and hope; the cultivation of sensitivity to one's self and to others; the development of a helping-trusting relationship; the promotion and acceptance of the expression of positive and negative feelings; the systematic use of the scientific problem-solving method; the promotion of interpersonal teaching-learning; the provision for a supportive, protective, and corrective mental, physical, sociocultural, and spiritual environment; the assistance with the gratification of human needs; and the allowance for existential-phenomenological forces. These caring factors can be viewed as providing a philosophical foundation for a model of caring for nursing education. More specifically, they suggest further organizational structure for caring interactions and transactions.

In her later work, Watson (1985) develops a theory of human caring based on her concept of transpersonal caring. She discusses the nature and value of caring as "a starting point . . . an attitude, which has to become a will, an intention, a commitment, and a conscious judgment that manifests itself in concrete acts" (p. 32). She argues that caring as a disciplinary value depends on the teaching of a caring ideology, requiring interpersonal demonstration and practice.

King (1981) proposes that all nursing actions are characterized by goal-oriented interactions and transactions between a nurse and a client in an active, helping process. A transactional process involves the sharing of values, goals, ideas, and knowledge that leads to advanced growth and development and mutual goal attainment.

These nursing theorists describe relationships between a nurse and one who is nursed. As a discipline attempts to develop and organize a body of knowledge, congruency between models and theories for practice *and* education becomes a major goal. Existing nursing theory provides further direction and support for the development of a caring model for nursing education.

Support from Nursing Studies. Philosophical analysis and concept development has described caring as a complex construct involving intention and action (Gaut, 1979), a preunderstanding of the ideology of nursing (Griffin, 1983), and as a motivating life force (Bevis, 1981). Gaut (1979, 1983, 1984) proposes that caring is a complex series of actions, an intentional process. Conditions for the action of caring to occur include regard, respect, knowledge, intention related to need, and positive change condition. Gaut's work has significant implications for the development of a caring model for nursing education. She provides a pathway for further analysis of the complex nature of caring interactions and transactions.

Clinical investigations of caring in nursing practice have looked at perceptual aspects of caring in the nurse-client dyad. Brown (1986) and Reiman (1986), in phenomenological studies, described patterns and structures of caring interactions from patients' perspectives. Experiences of care include such variables as existential, presence, recognition of individuality, confirmation, and listening-responding behaviors. These researchers urge the inclusion of existential philosophical thought in undergraduate nursing education.

Wolf (1986) developed a caring behavior inventory of 97 words and phrases that represent caring. Seventy-five registered nurses rankordered indicators of caring from their practice perspectives. Behaviors and attitudes chosen as most representative of caring included attentive listening, comforting, honesty, patience, and responsibility. Wolf calls for further investigation and documentation of the interactive behaviors that hallmark caring.

A number of studies have investigated the concept of empathy as an isolated indicator of effective caring interactions. Kalish (1971a, 1971b) described a course in empathy training for seniors in an associate degree program. Rosendahl (1973) investigated the concepts of empathy, nonpossessive warmth, and genuineness as they related to the self-actualization of nursing students. Stetler (1977) found a positive correlation between perceived empathy and the communication skill levels of senior nursing students. Blackburn (1982) reported that human relations training in empathic understanding, self-concept, and clinical performance were positively correlated in a group of sophomore nursing students. LaMonica (1983) described the development of an empathy training program using role-playing. These researchers incorporated humanistic and existential perspectives into their conceptual frameworks. They verify the importance of an interactional process in the education of nursing students.

Bush's research (1988) identifies six major concepts that constitute a model of the caring teacher in nursing. They include: knowledge and love of self and others, presence, mutual respect, sensitivity, communication with the other, and the organization of the teaching-learning situation. Bush argues that before a student can understand a person who needs care, knowledge of the self as a caring person must be developed. The person giving care needs to be caring before attempting to care for another. The nurse educator, by being an exemplar of care, can develop a caring posture in the nursing student. The six concepts identified by Bush provide further organizational structure for caring indicators and concepts. A caring model for nursing education as an interpersonal process affirms the importance of exemplar attitudes and activities on the part of the NE. Caring interactions and transactions between the NE and the NS go beyond this perspective, however, and include an evolutionary process whereby both the NE and the NS come to an expanded knowledge of self as carer.

Summary of the Literature Support. A review, analysis, and synthesis of the literature provided an inventory of related concepts and subconcepts for model development. It was then necessary to specify the direction of the relationships or the organizational structure that they represent (Newman, 1979). This process incorporates both objective and subjective meanings of caring.

Structural Refinement of the Model

Three structures were developed to organize the concepts and subconcepts. They represent the critical elements or "meaning spaces" of the constructs, caring interactions, and caring transactions proposed in the model. These are seen in Tables 1, 2, and 3.

The development of caring consciousness implies that the first stage of the interpersonal caring process depends upon a knowledge of the "I," or man's place in the world and how he relates to it. This structure can be conceived of as a caring for the self.

The development of caring mutuality incorporates attitudinal perspectives of an "I-thou" relationship, and implies a caring for the other in mutual growth processes.

The development of caring exchanges includes mutual caring activities and builds on elements in the first two structures. The process is

Table 1
Development of
Caring Consciousness

Attention to—concern for

Availability

Consciousness

Presence

Table 2
Development of
Caring Mutuality

Acceptance	Participation
Attachment	Positive regard
Concern	Prizing
Confirmation	Realness
Empathy	Respect
Genuineness	Responsibility
Honesty	Self-disclosure
Interest	Trust

Table 3
Development of Caring Exchanges

Adaptability	Facilitation
Assistance	Organization
Communication	Participation
Decision making	Problem solving

one of mutual growth and change that develops over time, where both the NE and the NS move toward transformation.

AUXILIARY THEORY DEVELOPMENT

Definitions, linkages, and conceptual relationships are being investigated to establish auxiliary theoretical support for the proposed model (Newman, 1979). Using a descriptive, correlational design, the relationship between caring interactions, transactions, and transformation from the perspective of the student nurse is being examined. Is there a positive relationship between a NS's perceptions of caring interactions and transactions with a NE, and the growth and transformation of the NS?

Study Variables

The constructs chosen for study are the NS's perceptions of caring interactions and transactions with NEs, proposed as the predictor or antecedent variable, and the level of the NS's growth and transformation, proposed as the criterion or resultant variable. The following definitions have been developed.

Theoretical Definitions

Caring Interaction. Caring interaction incorporates attitudinal structures of an interpersonal caring process between NE and a NS. It is characterized by perceptions of positive regard, warmth, empathic understanding, congruence, self-disclosure and genuineness (Carkhuff, 1984; Rogers, 1969; Sheston, 1988a, 1988b).

Caring Transaction. Caring transaction incorporates activity related structures of an interpersonal caring process between a NE and a NS. It is characterized by a dialogical quality of existential awareness, congruent role expectations, mutual goal setting and responsibility, and mutual positive change (Gaut, 1979; King, 1981; Paterson & Zderad, 1988; Sheston, 1988a; Watson, 1985).

Transformation. Transformation is a process of evolutionary change and self-actualization experienced as a result of caring interactions and transactions in the academic environment. Transformation is characterized by a greater being, an increased awareness of individual human caring potential, and relatedness to others. It is a positive term for the positive process of negentropy and implies increasing levels of complexity and organization. (Buber, 1958; Maslow, 1970; Mayeroff, 1971; Putt, 1978; Sheston, 1988b; Watson, 1985, 1987).

While theoretical definitions provide the theoretical meaning spaces or the "why" of particular concepts and relationships, operational definitions attempt to locate the concepts using specific empirical indicators, providing the "how" for asserting particular relationships (Hage, 1972).

Operational Definitions

Caring Interactions and Transactions. These are the NS's perceptions of caring interactions and transactions with NEs as measured by the Barrett-Lennard Relationship Inventory (BLRI) (1962).

Transformation.   Transformation is the NS's level of growth and self-actualization as human carers as measured by the Personal Orientation Inventory (Shostrom, 1966).

Discussion of the Instruments

The most serious problem in doing research on complex behavioral constructs is establishing the validity of the empirical measures used for theoretical and logical fit. Using and refining such instruments is a gradual process. Relationships between the theory and constructs being tested and the validity of the measurement tools evolve gradually (Layton, 1979).

The Barrett-Lennard Relationship Inventory (BLRI) (1962) measures the perceptions of an individual involved in a meaningful interpersonal relationship. The instrument includes subscales of unconditionality of regard, level of regard, empathy, and congruence. Concepts of empathic understanding, warmth, trust, validation, and genuineness are included. The BLRI has been found to have content, predictive, and construct validity as a measurement of the personal experience of understanding assessed by an individual in an interpersonal framework (Barrett-Lennard, 1962; Caracena & Victory, 1969; Kurtz & Grummon, 1972; Truax, 1966). These authors also provide sufficient evidence to support reliability, both split-half and test-retest in ranges of .82 to .95 with diverse populations. Alves, Bahiense, and Michael (1979) tested the validity of a unitary construct with the BLRI and concluded that the four subscales of unconditionality of regard, level of regard, empathy, and congruence contributed individually to the validation of the theory behind the construct of interpersonal relationship.

The Personal Orientation Inventory (POI) (Shostrom, 1966) attempts to measure the development of self-actualization and personal growth. The instrument consists of two basic scales and ten subscales, and includes concepts related to personal development, interpersonal interaction, existentiality, awareness of man, self-regard, and sensitivity to self and others. Reliability coefficients range from .55 to .85, and normative data for content validity is good, based on 2,607 college freshmen (Shostrom, 1966). Bloxom (1978) reports a high degree of validity for the instrument as a measure of feelings, values, and attitudes appropriate to self-actualization; convergent validity has been established by positive correlations to tests of empathy and facilitative genuineness in education students, and to ratings of teachers' concern for their students. Bloxom does mention pervasive overlapping with the instrument's subscales, but remarks that the two major scales are free of this problem. Coan (1978) concurs with this critique, and adds that positive intercorrelations among the scales are in accord with theoretical expectations. He encourages further clarification through research. Martin, Blair, Rudolf, and Melman (1981) estimated intercorrelations among the scales for 89 nursing students and found larger correlations than those reported in the manual as well as by others. Hattie (1986) reviewed the psychometric properties of the POI and concluded that it can be reasonably and meaningfully used as an assessment of personal growth.

Summary of Empirical Investigation

A descriptive measurement of theoretical constructs looks at degrees of relationships and attempts to measure facts and characteristics of a given population or area of interest (Isaac & Michael, 1981). The purpose of this study is to explain the nature of the relationship between the variables. The emphasis is on explanation of the variability of a criterion variable (student transformation) by using information from the predictor variable (student perceptions of caring interactions and transactions) (Waltz & Bausell, 1981). Since the study is designed to identify and describe variables that are theorized as components of a complex behavioral pattern, data will be analyzed by correlating these measures at the same time (Borg & Gall, 1983).

CONCLUSION

Disciplines evolve out of a distinctive perspective and context, requiring a determination of the phenomena of interest and the questions that are posed (Donaldson & Crowley, 1978). Caring provides the central and unifying focus for the development of the knowledge and practices of nursing, and is nursing's blueprint for transforming the profession, the health care system, and society (Moccia, 1988b; Watson, 1987). It is essential that the further development of caring knowledge start with the process of nursing education. A caring model for nursing education establishes a starting point for transforming a new generation of nurses and establishing an evolutionary and expanded caring consciousness for the discipline and for humanity.

REFERENCES

Alves, A., Bahiense, V., & Michael, W. (1979). Empirical test of the validity of unitary construct underlying a modified form of the Barrett-Lennard Relationship Inventory. *Educational and Psychological Measurement, 39*(2), 499–504.

Barrett-Lennard, G. T. (1962). *Dimensions of therapist response as casual factors in therapeutic change. Psychological Monologs*, No. 562, *76*(43).

Barrett, W. (1962). *Irrational man.* New York: Doubleday.

Bevis, E. O. (1981). Caring: a life force. In M. Leininger (Ed.), *Caring: An essential human need* (pp. 49–59). Thorofare, NJ: Slack.

Bevis, E. O. (1988). New directions for a new age. In *Curriculum revolution: Mandate for change.* New York: NLN Publications.

Blackburn, D. A. (1982). *The effect of human relations training on empathic understanding, self-concept and the clinical performance of sophomore student nurses.* Unpublished doctoral dissertation, Ball State University, Muncie, IN.

Blalock, H. M. (1969). *Theory construction: from verbal to mathematical formulations.* Englewood Cliffs, NJ: Prentice-Hall.

Bloxom. (1978). Review of Personal Orientation Inventory. In *Buros Mental Measurements Yearbook* (7th ed.). Highland Park, NJ: Gryphon Press.

Borg, W. R. & Gall, M. D. (1983). *Educational research: An introduction* (4th ed.). New York: Longman.

Brown, L. (1986). The experience of care. Patient perspectives. *Topics in Clinical Nursing, 8,* 84–93.

Buber, M. (1958). *I and thou* (3d ed.) (R. G. Smith, Ed. & Trans.). New York: Scribner.

Bush, H. (1988). The caring teacher of nursing. In M. Leininger (Ed.), *Care: Discovery and Uses in Clinical and Community Nursing.* Detroit: Wayne State University Press.

Caracena, P., & Vicory, J. (1969). Correlates of phenomenological and judged empathy. *Journal of Counseling Psychology, 16*(6), 510–515.

Carkhuff, R. R. (1969). *Helping and human relations: A primer for lay and professional helpers,* Vols. 1 & 2. New York: Holt, Rinehart & Winston.

Coan, R. W. (1978). Review of Personal Orientation Inventory. In *Buros Mental Measurements Yearbook* (7th ed.). Highland Park, NJ: Gryphon Press.

Donaldson, S., & Crowley, D. (1978). The discipline of nursing. *Nursing Outlook,* 26, 113–120.

Fromm, E. (1962). *The art of loving.* New York: Bantam Books.

Gaut, D. (1979). An application of the Kerr-Soltis model to the concept of caring in nursing education. *Dissertation Abstracts International, 40,* 6A (University Microfilms No. 79-27790).

Gaut, D. (1983). Development of a theoretically adequate description of caring. *Western Journal of Nursing Research, 5,* 313–24.

Gaut, D. (1984). A theoretical description of caring as action. In M. M. Leininger (Ed.), *Caring: The Essence of Nursing and Health* (pp. 27–44). Thorofare, NJ: Slack.

Griffin, A. P. (1983). A philosophical analysis of caring in nursing. *Journal of Advanced Nursing, 8,* 289–295.

Hage, J. (1972). *Techniques and problems in theory construction in sociology.* New York: Wiley.

Hattie, J. (1986). A defense of the Shostrom personal orientation inventory: A rejoinder to Ray. *Personality & Individual Differences, 7*(4), 593–594.

Isaac, S. & Michael, W. B. (1981). *Handbook in research and evaluation* (2d ed.). San Diego: Edits Publishers.

Jones, R. (1941). *Spirit in man.* Stanford: Stanford University Press.

Kalish, B. (1971a). An experiment in the development of empathy in nursing students. *Nursing Research, 20*(3), 202–211.

Kalish, B. (1971b). Strategies for developing nurse empathy. *Nursing Outlook, 19*(11), 714–718.

Kine, I. (1981). *A theory for nursing. Systems, concepts, process.* New York: Wiley.

Kurtz, R. R. & Grummon, D. L. (1972). Different approaches to the measurement of therapist empathy and their relationship to therapy outcomes. *Journal of Clinical Psychology, 39,* 106–113.

LaMonica, E. (Summer, 1983). Empathy can be learned. *Nurse Educator, 8*(9), 19–23.

Layton, J. M. (1979). The use of modeling to teach empathy to student nurses. *Research in Nursing and Health, 2,* 163–176.

Leininger, M. M. (March 1977). The phenomenon of caring: Caring, the essence and critical focus of nursing. *American Nurses' Foundation Nursing Research Report, 2*(14).

Leininger, M. M. (1978). *Transcultural nursing: Concepts, theories, practices.* New York: Wiley.

Leininger, M. M. (1984). *Care: The essence of nursing and health.* Thorofare, NJ: Slack.

Marcel, G. (1971). *The philosophy of existence* (R. F. Grabow, Ed. & Trans.). Philadelphia: University of Pennsylvania Press.

Martin, J., Blair, G., Rudolph, L., & Melman, B. (1981). Intercorrelations among scale scores of the personal orientation inventory for nursing students. *Psychological Reports, 48*(1), 199–202.

Maslow, A. H. (1970). *Motivation and personality* (2d ed.). New York: Harper & Row.

May, R. (1969). *Love and will.* New York: Norton.

Mayeroff, M. (1971). *On caring.* New York: Harper & Row.

Mead, G. H. (1934). *Mind, self and society.* Chicago: University of Chicago Press.

Moccia, P. (1988a). Curriculum revolution: An agenda for change. In *Curriculum revolution: Mandate for change.* New York: National League for Nursing.

Moccia, P. (1988b). At the faultline: Social activism and caring. *Nursing Outlook, 36*(1), 30–33.

Newman, M. A. (1979). *Theory development in nursing.* Philadelphia: Davis.

Paterson, J. G., & Zderad (1988). *Humanistic nursing.* New York: National League for Nursing.

Peplau, H. E. (1952). *Interpersonal relations in nursing.* New York: Putnam.

Putt, A. M. (1978). *General systems theory applied to nursing.* Boston: Little, Brown.

Rieman, D. J. (1986). The essential structure of a caring interaction: Doing phenomenology. In P. L. Munchall & C. J. Oiler (Eds.), *Nursing research: A qualitative perspective* (pp. 85–105). Norwalk, CT: Appleton-Century-Crofts.

Rogers, D. (1951). *Client-centered therapy: Its current practice, implications and theory.* Boston: Houghton-Mifflin.

Rogers, C. (1957). The necessary and sufficient conditions of therapeutic personality change. *Journal of Consulting Psychology, 21,* 95–103.

Rogers, C. (1961). *On becoming a person.* Boston: Houghton-Mifflin.

Rogers, C. (1965). *Client-centered therapy.* Boston: Houghton-Mifflin.

Rogers, C. (1969). *Freedom to learn.* Columbus: Merrill.

Rogers, C. (1975). Empathic. An unappreciated way of being. *The Counseling Psychologist, 5*(2), 2–10.

Rosendahl, P. (1973). Effectiveness of empathy, non-possessive warmth, and genuineness on self-actualization of students. *Nursing Research, 22*(3), 253–257.

Sheston, M. L. (1988a). *Caring in nursing education. The development of a construct.* Paper presented at the Tenth National Caring Conference. Boca Raton, FL: Florida Atlantic University.

Sheston, M. L. (1988b). *Caring in nursing education: A conceptual model.* Unpublished manuscript. Chester, PA: Widener University School of Nursing.

Shostrom, E. L. (1966). *Actualizing assessment battery, personal orientation inventory*. San Diego: Edits Publishers.

Stetler, C. (1977). Relationship of perceived empathy to nurses' communication. *Nursing Research, 26*(6), 432–438.

Truax, C. B. (1966). Therapist empathy, warmth, and genuineness and patient personality change in group psychotherapy: A comparison between interaction unit measures, time sample measures, patient perception measures. *Journal Clinical Psychology, 22,* 225–229.

Travelbee, J. (1971). *Interpersonal aspects of nursing* (2d ed.). Philadelphia: Davis.

Waltz, C. & Bausell, R. B. (1981). *Nursing research: Design, statistics, and computer analysis*. Philadelphia: Davis.

Watson, J. (1979). *Nursing: The philosophy and science of caring*. Boston: Little, Brown.

Watson, J. (1985). *Nursing: Human science and human care. A theory of nursing*. Norwalk, CT: Appleton-Century-Crofts.

Watson, J. (1987). Human caring and aging: A transcendent view. *Distinguished Lecture*. Washington, DC: Catholic University of America.

Wiedenbach, E. (1964). *Clinical nursing: A helping art*. New York: Springer-Verlag.

Wolf, Z. (1986). The caring concept and nurse-identified caring behaviors. *Topics in Clinical Nursing, 8,* 84–93.

10

The Experience of Caring in the Teaching-Learning Process of Nursing Education: Student and Teacher Perspectives

Barbara Krainovich Miller
Judith Haber
Mary Woods Byrne

Caring has been an integral part of nursing since the days of Nightingale. According to Watson (1985b), "human care is the heart of nursing" (p. 346). Although nursing's tradition indicated that caring was one of its essential values, caring has not been clearly described in nursing theories, nursing practice, or nursing education (Watson, 1985a, 1988). Although caring is considered essential to the teaching-learning process, little research exists as to what exactly constitutes caring in the educational setting. Some research has been reported on the phenomenon of caring in relation to nurses and patients (Warren, 1989).

The caring movement in nursing is led by Watson (1985a, 1985b, 1987) and Leininger (1981, 1984). Acts of caring are "essential for human development, growth, and survival" (Leininger, 1981, p. 11). At times caring has been undervalued in both nursing and nursing education, perhaps due in large part to the dominant male paradigm for the development of knowledge and curing the sick (Watson, 1988). Many in nursing education nevertheless have unknowingly followed the work of Mayeroff (1971). They are caring educators who "encourage and further it [caring] in others [students and clients]" (Mayeroff, 1971, p. 52). However, little research exists as to what exactly constitutes caring in the clinical setting. It is therefore essential to know how students experience caring so that caring experiences can be provided.

PURPOSE AND RESEARCH QUESTION

The purpose of this qualitative study was to add to nursing's body of knowledge related to the phenomenon of caring. The specific aim was to add to the understanding of the phenomenon of educational caring by asking students and teachers to recall and describe an interaction involving caring in the teaching-learning process.

The following research question was asked: What is the lived experience of a caring teacher-learning interaction from the perspective of nursing students and nursing faculty?

METHODOLOGY

Design Overview

Phenomenological analysis as developed by Streubert (1989) and adapted from the works of Colaizzi (1978), Giorgi (1985), and Valle and King (1978) comprised the methodology of this study. Specifically, phenomenological analyses of open-ended interviews were conducted. The focus of the interviews with informants was to identify themes of caring in the teaching-learning interaction.

Data reliability was increased by the consistent use of a guide for conducting the open-ended interviews. Saturation of themes cued the researchers that sufficient data were collected. Three interviewers minimized the bias that each alone might bring to identification of themes. Confidentiality of the informants was maintained.

Subjects and Setting

A convenience and purposive sample of six senior nursing students and six nursing faculty, who had taught for at least three years, volunteered to participate in the study. The setting was a small liberal arts college department of nursing in the metropolitan area of a large eastern city of the United States. The interviews were conducted in a well-ventilated, acoustically sound room that was familiar to the informants.

Instrument

Open-ended interviews were used by the investigators. An interview guide was developed so each of the three researchers would follow the suggested guidelines for encouraging the informant to explore thoughts on a caring interaction. Student informants were asked the following question: "Tell me about a caring teaching-learning interaction you have experienced during one of your nursing courses." Faculty informants were asked: "Tell me about a teaching-learning interaction in which you provided caring."

The researchers met prior to conducting the interviews and reviewed the interview guide protocol, determined the setting for the interviews, and role-played interviews with student and faculty. In addition, tape recorders with moveable microphones were secured; tapes and recorder were pretested in the designated interview room.

Procedure

The voluntary informants' names were randomly assigned to the three investigators. Informed consent as well as a date and time for the interview was obtained. In addition, informants were asked to dwell on a caring teaching-learning interaction prior to the interview.

At the time of the taped open interview the investigator:

1. Reviewed the study's purpose.
2. Reviewed the consent form and elicited the informants signature.
3. Initiated the interview by requesting that the student informant describe a situation in the teaching-learning process in which he/she experienced "caring" or requested that the faculty informant describe a situation in which he/she gave "caring."
4. Encouraged the informants to provide sufficient content for clarification.

After three interviews with students, themes and patterns related to caring emerged. However, three additional interviews with students were conducted to ensure that we had not ended the interviews too soon. Caring themes also emerged after three faculty interviews and a total of six were conducted.

ANALYSIS

Transcriptions of twelve audio-taped interviews were initially read by each researcher while listening to the audio tape to determine the accuracy of the transcriptions. One transcription was not usable. The 11 transcriptions were then reread to gain an understanding of their expressed feelings. Then caring statements were identified and transcribed to index cards. The three researchers then met to share and discuss these identified caring statements. After several meetings the agreed-upon caring statements from the 11 transcripts were merged and caring themes identified. Once the themes were identified the researchers wrote the exhaustive descriptions of the phenomenon of caring experienced by students and faculty during a teaching-learning interaction. The student and faculty informants were sent the respective descriptions for validation. They were asked if the written description captured the essence of their perception of a caring teaching-learning interaction.

FINDINGS

Themes

The four major themes derived from both the student and the faculty interviews were parallel: holistic concern or philosophy, teacher ways of being, mutual simultaneous dimensions, and student ways of being. These themes are reflected in the following exhaustive descriptions that the informants agreed captured the essence of a caring student-teacher interaction.

Student Description Of a Caring Teaching-Learning Interaction

Students describe the caring teaching-learning interaction as a process characterized by a pervasive climate of support whether it is in a one-to-one or group context. Within this climate of support, the process of caring develops. The process emerges out of a perceived need of the student that is anticipated or recognized by the teacher or a student concern/problem that is brought to the attention of the teacher by the student.

Students perceive that an essential dimension of the caring interaction is the faculty's holistic concern for the student, personally and academically. Students identify caring teachers as being nonjudgmental, respectful, patient, available, dependable, flexible, supportive, open, warm, and genuine.

They perceive that the teacher reaches out to them in an empathetic way offering a constant presence. Students describe the constant presence as the caring faculty member always being there for them. Caring faculty protect them from pitfalls in the clinical setting in relation to direct patient care as well as their academic grades while simultaneously enabling them to anticipate the reality of the situation so they often can cope beyond their own expectations. From this process students perceive that caring faculty recognize their underdeveloped and actual strengths in relation to personal and academic needs. Caring faculty provide feedback and help students to explore thoughts, feelings, and options. They are further described as empowering individuals who enable students to autonomously reach their personal and academic potentials.

Students perceive that caring interactions involve the mutual simultaneous dimensions of intimacy, connectedness, trust, sharing, and respect. In such interactions the caring teacher is perceived as one who goes beyond the "expected" teacher role and may even act as a friend.

Through the process of caring in a student/faculty interaction the relationship between the student and teacher is much stronger. Students relate that they experience movement toward self-actualization. They express experiencing increased self-worth, self-esteem, and self-confidence. They are able to recognize their own progress, which gives them faith in themselves and hope for the future. They say caring interactions leave them feeling good, happy, courageous, and proud.

For students, a caring interaction is more than just trusting and "all that stuff," it's like all those things added together without boundaries which is something bigger than the sum of its parts.

Faculty Description of a Caring Teaching-Learning Interaction

Faculty describe a caring teaching-learning interaction as an interactive process integral with a philosophical position about caring as the foundation of a student-teacher relationship. Caring emerges from this philosophical perspective and reflects the teacher's holistic view about students.

Faculty perceive that the teacher acts as a role model in the relationship with the student, mirroring the caring behaviors they expect will be assimilated by the student to be reflected in their patient interactions. The caring teacher reaches out to students with empathy, sensitivity, openness, warmth, and respect. Within a nonjudgmental climate of privacy and support, faculty validate students' feelings and self-worth while simultaneously recognizing their underdeveloped and actual strengths.

Teachers act as facilitators and resource persons who enable students to push toward increasing personal and professional autonomy. By providing unbounded availability, follow-up, and acceptance, they protect students from pitfalls while empowering them through encouragement of self-exploration, self-discovery, and expansion of perceptual boundaries.

Teachers perceive that caring interactions involve the mutual simultaneous dimensions of trust, respect, openness, reciprocity, sharing, acceptance, sincerity, and genuineness. The interactive process is initiated and continued through the use of effective verbal and nonverbal communication skills. It is a reciprocal process that becomes a learning experience for both faculty and students. As a result of the caring interaction, faculty describe feeling good, comfortable, effective, and, at times, motherly.

Faculty report that students describe that caring interactions make them feel better about themselves and better able to handle problematic situations. Faculty also report that students often contact them years later to tell them about the lasting value of a specific caring interaction. For faculty, caring is the essence of the student-teacher relationship. They say "If we don't care, how can we expect students to care?"

Discussion of Themes in Exhaustive Descriptions

Holistic Concern/Philosophy. Both students and faculty emphasized holistic regard for individuals as a fundamental quality of the phenomenon of caring. Students talked in detail about their intertwined academic and personal needs and how faculty responded to all of these needs in an individual manner. The researchers called this "holistic concern." Faculty labeled as "holistic philosophy" the paradigm through which they deliberately approached students.

The theme of holism is implicitly embedded in the caring literature, in particular, the evolving caring theories of Leininger (1981, 1984, 1985) and Watson (1979, 1985a), and the philosophical work of Mayeroff (1971). What is striking in the findings of this study is that the informants explicitly dwelled on the significance of a holistic perspective permeating the caring experience.

Teacher and Student Ways of Being.   The researchers identified the existential qualities of the sharers in the caring process and labeled these themes "teacher ways of being" and "student ways of being." Students stressed the dimensions of a climate of support and faculty specified strategies they consciously used to develop this climate. Both students and faculty identified empowerment, growth, and hope for the future as student outcomes of caring interactions with faculty.

These existential qualities are consistent with one of Watson's assumptions about caring; that is, that "caring attitudes allow a person to be as he/she is now but also to actualize potentialities for being different in the future" (1985a, p. 42). The characteristics described as student and teacher ways of being also reflect more than half the major taxonomic caring constructs of Leininger (1981). Riemen (1986) recommended that nursing educators should demonstrate "presence, really listening and respect for the uniqueness of the individual . . . so that students can know the receptivity of caring" (p. 104). These characteristics of the caring educator specifically emerged from the student and faculty interviews.

Mutual Simultaneous Dimensions.   Both faculty and students perceived caring in teaching-learning encounters as an ongoing and interactive process, a theme the researchers named "mutual simultaneous dimensions." Parallel subthemes of trust, sharing, and respect were expressed by students and faculty. However, while students emphasized the importance of intimacy and connectedness in the relationship, faculty focused on reciprocity and openness. In both cases the value of learning from each other was integral to the caring process.

The caring philosophy of Mayeroff (1971) supports the validity of the themes described as mutual simultaneous dimensions. In particular, Mayeroff (1971) stressed the mutuality of the one cared for and the caregiver with each learning from the other. Both are significant participants in a process of discovery; neither is too important to learn from the other.

IMPLICATIONS AND RECOMMENDATIONS

As the nursing profession continues to develop the body of knowledge specific to its science, in-depth understanding of the common essences of caring will help to enlighten and direct its future. Further description of the phenomenon of caring in relation to nursing education will help to explicate nursing's paradigm of the art of caring (Peplau, 1988). According to student nurse informants in a study by Byrne (1988), "caring" nursing education can be critical to the recruitment and retention of nursing students.

The results of our study on describing the phenomenon of caring in relation to the teaching-learning process add to nursing's knowledge and theories on caring in general. Specifically, knowledge has been generated on caring in relation to the educational setting. Such knowledge can be incorporated into the graduate curriculum of programs preparing nursing educators; integrated into undergraduate nursing curricula; used in faculty development and inservice nursing education programs; and borrowed by other disciplines for incorporation in their curricula. Such knowledge will assist faculty and inservice educators in their role modeling of caring behaviors to all levels of nursing students and nurses, thus maximizing their educational experiences. In turn, nursing students and nurses would have an increased ability to offer "caring" to their clients. As expressed by our faculty informants: "If we don't care, how can we expect them [students] to care?" In a similar vein, a student informant said: "It's like how they [faculty] are with us is how we should be with our patients."

Students and faculty described caring as a crucial dimension of the educational phenomenon. This suggests that caring as a curriculum foundation or thread should be more fully and clearly developed in nursing programs. Rather than relying solely on the individual teacher's caring philosophy, curriculum development related to caring should be based on emerging research findings. The new paradigm for nursing and nursing education advocates a moral context of health and human caring. Watson (1988) has envisioned a doctoral program based on human caring. Boykin (1989) has operationalized caring as the foundation of the nursing program at Florida Atlantic University. Our research findings reinforce the significance of continuing to move in this direction.

Faculty development programs are needed to teach faculty about the theory of caring and its place in undergraduate and graduate curriculum. Faculty development can also focus on strategies to enhance caring behaviors in both faculty and students and the extension of these behaviors to relationships with patients. For example, empathy can be one manifestation of caring that can be taught in communication workshops framed within a caring perspective.

Future research can also link the constructs comprising caring and clarify their relationships so that propositions can be stated and tested. For example, the relationship of empathy to the phenomenon of caring needs to be clarified. In this study empathy was identified as meaningful within each theme. Gadow (1988) states that it is the "intensity of empathic regard" that enables a nurse to engage in mutuality with a client and that empathy is an essential condition for care which emerges from the nurse's own vulnerability and allows the nurse to relate to the patient so that care and cure are synthesized. This dimension of mutuality also emerged in our study as a significant theme and a condition through which caring evolves in the teaching-learning process.

As additional research illuminates the phenomenon of caring in relation to empathy, mutuality and related constructs, the specifics of how to teach caring, how to learn it, and how to bring it into our practice will be more clearly defined. As the body of knowledge concerning caring grows, not only nursing but all "caring" professions can draw from it.

A unique aspect of our phenomenological study was the participation by three researchers in collecting, processing, and synthesizing the data. We met together for at least nine sessions ranging from two to six hours. It was during these sessions that we learned and lived a process of effective collaboration. We discovered that longer sessions of three to six hours were most productive, and allowed for a "dwelling together with the data" in a way that enabled us to reach consensus on the patterns of meaning enveloped in the numerous statements that had been identified as significant. We were committed to talking out the meaning each of us inferred from a particular "caring statement" to achieve clarification and consensus.

Our collaborative analysis sessions were marked by a sense of mutual respect; by patience with ourselves, with each other, and with the complexity of the data; and with a sense of humor that paradoxically enabled us to attend to our seriousness of purpose. We encourage other researchers to collaborate in their research endeavors when using either the quantitative or qualitative methodology. The positive aspects of collaborative studies far outweigh any negative aspects one might encounter.

REFERENCES

Byrne, M. (1988). *An ethnography of undergraduate nursing students' clinical learning field.* Doctoral dissertation, Adelphi University, Garden City, NY. (UMI No. 8814972).

Colaizzi, P. F. (1978). Psychological research as the phenomenologist views it. In R. Valle & M. King (Eds.), *Existential-phenomenological alternatives for psychology.* New York: Oxford University Press.

Gadow, S. (1988). Covenant without cure: Letting go and holding on in chronic illness. In J. Watson & M. Ray (Eds.), *The ethics of care and the ethics of cure: Synthesis in chronicity.* New York: National League for Nursing.

Giorgi, A. (1985). *Phenomenology and psychological research.* Pittsburgh, PA: Duquesne University Press.

Leininger, M. M. (1981). *Caring: An essential human need.* Thorofare, NJ: Slack.

Leininger, M. M. (1984). *Caring: The essence of nursing and health.* Thorofare, NJ: Slack.

Leininger, M. M. (1985). Ethnography and Ethnonursing: Models and modes of qualitative data analysis. In M. M. Leininger (Ed.), *Qualitative research methods in nursing* (pp. 33–71). Orlando, FL: Grune & Stratton.

Mayeroff, M. (1971). *On caring.* New York: Harper & Row.

Olesen, V. & Whittaker, E. (1968). *The silent dialogue.* San Francisco: Jossey-Bass.

Peplau, H. E. (1988). The art and science of nursing: Similarities, differences, and relations. *Nursing Science Quarterly, 1*(1), 8–15.

Riemen, D. (1986). The essential structure of a caring interaction: Doing phenomenology. In P. Munhall & C. J. Oiler, (Eds.), *Nursing research: A qualitative perspective* (pp. 85–108). Norwalk, CT: Appleton-Century-Crofts.

Streubert, H. J. (1989). *A description of clinical experience as perceived by clinical nurse educators and students.* Unpublished doctoral dissertation, Teachers College, Columbia University.

Valle, R. S., & King, M. (1978). *Existential phenomenological alternatives for psychology.* New York: Oxford Press.

Warner, L. (1989). Review and synthesis of 9 nursing studies on care and caring. *Journal of New York State Nurses Association, 19*(4), 10–16.

Watson, J. (1979). *Nursing: The philosophy and science of care.* Boston: Little, Brown.

Watson, J. (1985a). *Nursing: A human science and human care. A theory of nursing.* Norwalk, CT: Appleton-Century-Crofts.

Watson, J. (1985b). Reflecting on different methodologies for the future of nursing. In M. M. Leininger (Ed.), *Qualitative research in methods in nursing* (pp. 343–349). Orlando, FL: Grune & Stratton.

Watson, J. (1987). *Nursing on the caring edge: Metaphorical vignettes.* Rockville, MD: Aspen.

Watson, J. (1988). Human caring as moral context for nursing education. *Nursing & Health Care, 9*(8), 422–425.

11

Make Room for Care: Challenges for Faculty of Undergraduate Nursing Curricula

Mary Ellen Symanski

It is heartening to see that care is receiving such enthusiastic attention among nursing scholars. We must convey this enthusiasm to our next generation of nurses. I believe that to teach care meaningfully and effectively, care must be central in the curriculum. In this regard, several key issues must be addressed. First, do faculty know what they mean by care? Scholars looking at care conceptualize it in diverse ways; how faculty implement teaching care in the curriculum will reflect these conceptualizations and perhaps others of their own. Second, how do we make room to teach care. Already there are many demands from the health care system on faculty preparing basic nursing practitioners.

WHAT IS CARE?

I will examine several ways that care has been viewed, how these perspectives have been implemented in nursing curricula, and present suggestions for new approaches to make care a more central focus in undergraduate nursing education.

Care as the Art of Nursing

One way of looking at care is in terms of the expressive interpersonal acts of nursing. Comforting, touching, and being with another person are examples of this type of care. By some, they are thought to represent the artistic dimensions of nursing practice (Henderson, 1988). Jean Watson, although opposed to dichotomizing the art and science of nursing, describes transpersonal caring as an art (1981, 1988). Paterson and Zderad's *Humanistic Nursing* also represents a perspective on caring which emphasizes interpersonal dimensions (Paterson & Zderad, 1988; Watson, 1988).

The art of nursing is sometimes contrasted with traditional biophysical science. Caring is seen as a humanizing force, or providing a "high-touch" dimension to counterbalance the "high-tech" care (Henderson, 1985; Kelley, 1984; Leininger, 1981, 1984, 1986).

How much a part of the curriculum are strategies to teach the affective, interpersonal caring behaviors? Therapeutic communication, appropriate use of touch, and nurse-patient relationships are examples of topics that would receive heavy emphasis in the classroom and laboratory in this view of care. There is some evidence that role modeling can be effective in teaching humanistic interpersonal skills. Studies by Kalisch (1971), LaMonica (1983), and Layton (1979) have demonstrated the usefulness of teaching empathy through role modeling techniques.

Values and Attitudes

Care is also conceptualized as values and as attitudes. They are related to interpersonal care behaviors, but perhaps call for other types of educational approaches. Several nurse leaders have published their ideas about care values. Ray (1981) speaks of a care ideology in nursing that promotes growth in people, and views it as a form of love. Riemen (1986) characterizes caring as valuing others as human beings. Watson (1988) speaks of care values that encompass a moral commitment toward preserving human dignity.

Several approaches to foster care values have been implemented in nursing curricula. One strategy involves an increased focus on liberal arts and humanities subjects. The thesis behind this approach is that students who are exposed to subjects such as art, literature, history, music, and anthropology will have deeper appreciation of humanity in general, and greater respect for humans on a one-to-one level (Reed, 1987). This position is supported by the American Association of Colleges of Nursing (1987).

An alternative approach to teaching care values is a deliberate consideration of existing nursing educational processes that may foster uncaring values. This idea has surfaced repeatedly in the nursing and general educational literature (Bush, 1988; King & Gerwig, 1981; Mauksch, 1972; Noddings, 1984; Stein, 1986). Choosing alternative approaches in teaching such as consciously caring for students and incorporating them in decision-making processes are suggested by these authors. The teaching process itself thus becomes a tool for inculcating care values.

Care as Action

Gaut takes a different view of caring by suggesting that it necessarily includes an action component as well as the intention to care. Gaut explicitly states that good intentions are not enough. The notion of caring as action broadens and specifies the idea of what effective caring is to include: goal setting, choosing tactics to meet goals, implementation of these tactics with skill, and relatedness of the actions to positive changes in the ones being cared for (Gaut, 1983, 1986).

Teaching of caring in light of caring actions would encompass a broader range of topics, for instance, behavioral psychology principles to foster positive patient behaviors. Teaching psychomotor skills would also be in the realm of caring, for they are considered caring actions to bring about beneficial changes in the one being cared for. Looking at care from this perspective, it would behoove nursing faculty to teach skillful implementation of actions such as endotracheal suction, bed baths, and intravenous line insertion.

Care Linked with Knowledge

Knowledge about the structure and function of human beings, as well as biomedical and psychological treatment modalities, has also been considered by some as a part of care. Watson refers to knowledge of sciences and clinical topics as a presupposition for care (1988). The volume of this knowledge is quite extensive, which is not surprising given the complexity of human beings. Clinical content related to human beings in health and illness has traditionally been given top priority in undergraduate

curricula. "Knowing what one is doing" is a broadly interpreted statement that is sometimes equated with care. This notion has been validated
in several studies using empirical research methods (Cronin & Harrison,
1988; Grau, 1984; Larson, 1987). However, while knowledge about human beings related to health care science and technology expands
rapidly, what to exclude and include in nursing curricula does not seem
to be carefully considered.

Care as Substantive Phenomenon

Leininger has been instrumental in defining and explicating the
phenomenon of care. She stresses the need to know the people's ways
of caring, and to have in-depth knowledge of care as a phenomenon
(1978, 1981, 1983, 1988). Through ethnographic research more than
85 care constructs have been explicated in diverse cultural groups
(1988). Examples of these care constructs are involvement, touch, protection, stress alleviation, comfort, and advocacy. The knowledge
about care unearthed in this research points to the diversity and complexity of care as a concept, and the importance of cultural affiliations
to care patterns (1981, 1984, 1986, 1988). In my experience, this
knowledge of care as a phenomenon is not as heavily emphasized in
nursing curricula.

To conclude, I contend that in most nursing schools care is not the
most prominent central theme. Although many care constructs, such as
comfort, concern, and stress alleviation, are taught in some way, and
faculty may endeavor to promote care values, care is not as explicit in
the curriculum as it should be. In the Slevin and Harter study (1987),
only 8.5% of the schools reported that care was a major concept or
organizing theme. In my experience, students are taught some degree
of caring interpersonal skills, and much clinical knowledge about the
health care of human beings, but less about the philosophy of care,
cultural care, and the substance of care.

Certainly research is warranted to validate the ways that care is and
is not being taught in nursing programs. I believe a beginning step in
this endeavor is to validate the ways in which faculty view care and
caring. One may find that faculty believe they are teaching care simply
because "they care." Care and caring may be treated as a given. Faculty
may say, "Of course I teach care!" Therefore, a serious investigation of
the teaching of care requires systematically delving into the meanings
faculty ascribe to care, and how they describe implementing these notions of care in the curriculum.

INCREASING THE CARE
EMPHASIS IN NURSING EDUCATION

I propose several ways to approach increasing the emphasis on care in undergraduate nursing education. These changes involve early introduction to the philosophical and conceptual basis of care, framing clinical courses with related care constructs, and limiting the presentation of content on nursing and medical clinical topics to a reasonable amount that students are capable of learning thoroughly.

Introduce Care Early

I would offer a course in the very first year of nursing education on the philosophy and science of human care. This course would introduce students to the ideas of Mayeroff, Gaylin, Watson, Leininger, and others. By requiring this course first, a strong message would be sent to nursing students—that care is considered a crucial element of nursing.

A nursing course, "Human Care: Cultural Care Dimensions," in the following semester would also be offered. This course would emphasize the importance of culture as a variable in determining care expressions. In addition to discussing factual information about cultures, this course could promote students' awareness of their own cultural practices and values.

In the second year, the topic of caring relationships would be introduced using the works of such nurse-scholars as Peplau, Orlando, Watson, Parse, and others. The student at this stage would have a solid introduction to the central concept of care and a strong sense that care is a dominant theme in the nursing major.

Care Constructs to Frame Clinical Courses

Seminars on specific care constructs could be used effectively in a nursing curriculum to frame clinical courses within a perspective of care. Presently, many instances of caring action may be taught without expressly alluding to the link with care. For instance, students are taught to assess changes in physical condition, yet this is not taught as surveillance. Students are taught to maintain a safe environment, yet this is not necessarily presented as protection.

Seminars on the care constructs would present knowledge about the constructs gained from research and examples of use of the constructs in clinical practice situations. For instance, presence, support, and advocacy could be emphasized when students are studying chronically ill and dying patients. In these seminars, offered concurrently with clinical courses, students would gain knowledge of care as a powerful therapeutic mode. They would understand that there is substantive knowledge to be learned about care. They would gain a nursing outlook on actions they perform in the clinical area. Most important, the message would be conveyed that excellence in nursing is centered around care.

MAKE ROOM FOR CARE

To make room for care, something must be given up. My proposal for one possible curriculum is one which limits care clinical competencies to those related to care of the adult client. The student would have the opportunity to choose one additional practice area in the senior year, such as maternal newborn care, critical care, care of the ill child, or home care. I contend that it is no longer possible to be competent in all areas that have been traditionally taught.

It may be difficult to convince faculty that limiting coverage of the traditional specialties may be the best option. The benefits to nursing students, however, would be far-reaching. First and foremost, students would be freed for the study of care. Second, students would feel more self-confident, as their knowledge of adult health care would be comprehensive rather than sketchy. It seems obvious that a nurse who is not overwhelmed in a practice setting will be more likely to express creativity in caring.

I have suggested several approaches to make care a dominant theme in nursing curricula. The changes I propose would require some change in both National League for Nursing accreditation and the basic licensure examination. Thus, in a way, the proposals may be viewed as radical. On the other hand, the concept of care could drive the curriculum in an even more unified way. There may be more changes in store for the entire health care system when nurse researchers, practicing nurses, and faculty gain a deeper understanding of the depth and breadth of the phenomenon of care. The proposed curriculum ideas are not meant to be a rigid mandate, rather a seed from which other ideas will grow. At present, I believe that any increase in the emphasis on care is a step in the right direction.

REFERENCES

AACN (1987). The essentials of college and university education for professional nursing. *Journal of Professional Nursing, 3*(1), 54–56.

Bush, H. A. (1988). The caring teacher of nursing. In M. Leininger (Ed.), *Care: Discovery and uses in clinical and community nursing.* Detroit, MI: Wayne State University Press.

Cronin, S. N., & Harrison, B. (1988). Importance of nurse caring behaviors as perceived by patients after myocardial infarction. *Heart and Lung, 17*(4), 374–380.

Gaut, D. A. (1983). Development of a theoretically adequate description of caring. *Western Journal of Nursing Research, 5*(4), 313–324.

Gaut, D. A. (1986). Evaluating care competencies in nursing practice. *Topics in Clinical Nursing, 8*(2), 77–83.

Grau, L. (1984). What older adults expect from the nurse. *Geriatric Nursing, 5,* 14–18.

Henderson, V. (1985). The essence of nursing in high technology. *Nursing Administration Quarterly, 9*(4), 1–9.

Kalisch, B. J. (1971). An experiment in the development of empathy in nursing students. *Nursing Research, 20*(2), 202–211.

Kelly, L. S. (1988). The ethic of caring: Has it been discarded? *Nursing Outlook, 36*(1), 17.

King, V., & Gerwig, N. (1981). *Humanizing nursing education: A confluent approach through group process.* Wakefield, MA: Nursing Resources.

LaMonica, E. (1983). Empathy can be learned. *Nurse Educator, 8,* 19–22.

Larson, P. (1984). Important nurse caring behaviors perceived by patients with cancer. *Oncology Nursing Forum, 11*(6), 46–50.

Layton, J. M. (1979). The use of modeling to teach empathy to nursing students. *Research in Nursing and Health, 2,* 163–176.

Leininger, M. M. (1981). The phenomena of caring: Importance, research questions, and theoretical considerations. In M. M. Leininger (Ed.), *Caring: An essential human need.* Thorofare, NJ: Slack.

Leininger, M. M. (1983). Cultural care: An essential goal for nursing and health. *American Association for Nephrology Nurses and Technicians, 10*(5), 11–17.

Leininger, M. M. (1984). Caring: A central focus of nursing in health care services. In M. M. Leininger (Ed.), *Care: The essence of nursing and health.* Thorofare, NJ: Slack.

Leininger, M. M. (1986). Care facilitation and resistance factors in the culture of nursing. *Topics in Clinical Nursing, 8*(2), 1–12.

Leininger, M. M. (1988). Leininger's theory of nursing: Cultural care diversity and universality. *Nursing Science Quarterly, 1*(4), 152–160.

Mauksch, I. G. (1972). Let's listen to the students. *Nursing Outlook, 24*(7), 441–445.

Noddings, N. (1984). *Caring: A physical approach to ethics and moral education.* Berkeley, CA: University of California Press.

Paterson, J. G., & Zderad, L. T. (1988). *Humanistic nursing.* New York: National League for Nursing.

Ray, M. A. (1981). A philosophical analysis of caring within nursing. In M. Leininger (Ed.), *Caring: An essential human need.* Thorofare, NJ: Slack.

Reed, P. G. (1987). Liberal arts and professional nursing education: Integrating knowledge and wisdom. *Nurse Educator, 12*(4), 37–40.

Riemen, D. J. (1986). Noncaring and caring in the clinical setting: Patients' descriptions. *Topics in Clinical Nursing, 8*(2), 56–62.

Slevin, A. P., & Harter, M. O. (1987). The teaching of caring: A survey report. *Nurse Educator, 12*(6), 23–26.

Stein, A. P. (1986). Teaching nurses to care. *Nurse Educator, 11*(6), 4.

Watson, J. (1981). Nursing's scientific quest. *Nursing Outlook, 29*(7), 413–416.

Watson, J. (1988). *Nursing: Human science and human care.* New York: National League for Nursing.

12

Knowing Care in the Clinical Field Context: An Educator's Point of View

Sharie Metcalfe

Nursing cannot abdicate its responsibility to deliver health care in a technological environment. Rather, its mandate is to care in a technological environment. This goal cannot be achieved by separating care into doing and being, instrumental and affective, or knowing and doing. It can only be realized by practicing the essence of caring in clinical skill. The premise of this chapter is that professional nurse caring is best demonstrated through clinical competence, which is knowledge and technical skill, and is taught only through planned clinical experience. This chapter is based on three interrelated ideas: generic care and professional care (Leininger, 1980); the contextual and cultural aspects of care and caring; and the primacy of the clinical field to know nursing (Reilly & Oermann, 1985).

TYPES OF CARING

The use of the constructs *generic care, professional care,* and *professional nursing care* are indispensable in facilitating the beginning student's comprehension of nurse caring. While these terms need continued development and research, they will still assist the learner in distinguishing how nurse caring differs from parent caring or teacher caring. This difference is crucial if students are to recognize a body of knowledge integral to professional nurse caring. Intuitive feelings and compassion are necessary but not sufficient for the professional nurse.

In all situations of human care, the caring agent expresses concern and engages in action to enhance the recipient's well-being. Generic caring is those assistive, supportive, or facilitative acts toward another to improve a human condition or lifeway (Leininger, 1981b). Hult (1980) describes this caring as an attentive concern. A parent's care for a child or the heartfelt concern of one friend for another are examples of generic care. Likewise, so is the support of a husband for his wife during labor or the involvement of a peer counselor during a support group meeting. These examples of a type of humanistic care illustrate concern with emotional response and recognition of the uniqueness of the individual. The responses of the care agent are intuitive. Generic care is the foundation of professional care but the structural elements and function of the caregiver and recipient differ (Leininger, 1980).

Professional care adds the component of scientific caring, those tested or known activities and judgments used in assisting an individual or group (Leininger, 1981a). In providing professional care, the caring agent demonstrates deliberate actions based on a circumscribed body of knowledge as a means to assist the recipient. Social workers and educators are examples of professions that claim ownership of a type of professional care (Noddings, 1984; Wilson, 1986).

Professional nurse caring is founded on professional care and is humanistic and scientific (Leininger, 1980, p. 136). Moreover, professional nursing care is distinct and different from generic care. It recognizes that a set of learned actions, techniques, and processes exists which can be communicated to the learner and the client. These modes of care are directed toward sustaining and improving the health and well-being of clients (Leininger, 1988). Because nursing is a practice discipline, the concept of professional nursing care is central to knowing care through clinical practice. That care and caring can be learned and requires practice is also supported by students of care in other disciplines. Mayeroff (1971) underscored this view by seeing caring as a growth toward self-actualization in which *knowledge* is focal. Noddings (1984) and other educators encouraged the *practice* of caring as a moral guide for teachers and students (Crisci, 1981; Fantini, 1980). Thus, Leininger's assumption of professional nurse care as cognitively learned behavior that can be transmitted is the basis for discovering and teaching caring in the clinical field context.

CONTEXTUAL AND CULTURAL ASPECTS OF CARING

Growing empirical evidence exists to support the premise that caring is cultural and contextual and professional nurses do not always know those caring behaviors and processes which clients value. Leininger (1984) found that rural blacks did not value modern technology in health care practices but placed a high value on touching. Whites, on the other hand, valued technology but rarely mentioned touching as a mode of caring. Watson (1988) reported finding differences in caring during loss-grieving experiences among Australian Anglo-Saxons and aborigines. Aamodt (1984) generated 20 cultural themes that described aspects of care and caring. Nurses' perceptions of nursing care behaviors also varied by culture. Asian nurses viewed talking with the client and family as less important than Caucasians. Asian nurses valued personal delivery of care more than Caucasians or blacks (Servellen, 1988). Analysis of caring by gender shows that females appreciate verbal caring more than men who value technical competence more (Henry, 1975; Weiss, 1984).

Contextual aspects of caring are also documented. Larson (1984, 1987) and Mayer (1986, 1987) investigated cancer patients' perceptions of nurse caring behaviors and found that competency in technical skills and nursing knowledge were highly valued by these patients. Cronin and Harrison (1988) identified professional competence, monitoring, and technical skill as most significant to myocardial infarction patients in critical care. Consistent with these finding were reports of Brown (1986), Watson, Burckhardt, Brown, Bloch, and Hester (1979), and Allanach and Golden (1988). Adult medical-surgical patients rank scientific-instrumental and "doing-for" activities above those in the affective domain.

In another study, psychiatric patients placed more emphasis on moral support, problem solving, and sharing feelings than did medical or surgical patients (Gardner & Wheeler, 1981). Surgical patients emphasized physical comfort activities. In a group of women experiencing pregnancy loss Swanson-Kauffman (1986) found that subjects identified knowing, being with, and doing for as caring.

As a group, nurses tend to be rather consistent in selecting listening as the priority caring behavior (Gardner & Wheeler, 1981; Larson, 1986;

Mayer, 1987; Wolf, 1986). Other nurse caring behaviors identified by nurses are empathy and concern, allowing patient to express feelings, and being available (Bowman, 1987; Gardner & Wheeler, 1981). Nurses do not identify technical skill and professional knowledge as caring behaviors as frequently as clients. This finding may result from gender difference, cultural influence, or professional socialization.

These and similar studies indicate that the meaning of care and caring varies from culture to culture and nursing situation to nursing situation and that nurses are not always aware of the client's perception of caring behaviors. Therefore, it is maintained that the clinical field context is critical to learning caring.

The use of the term "clinical field" has been suggested by Reilly and Oermann (1985) to represent the actual area of practice that involves patient contact. The clinical field provides a dynamic environment and a gestalt that contributes to the learner experiencing the practice of nursing and specifically the practice of caring. Nursing and nurse educators too frequently ignore the fact that nursing skills include a motor component, a cognitive component, an affective component, and a cultural component. When all are skillfully synthesized in care competence, it is a demonstration of professional nurse caring.

EXPERIENTIAL LEARNING IN THE CLINICAL FIELD

My pedagogical approach to teach caring is based on Gestalt learning theory, Hergenhahn's theory (1982) that one experiences before learning and a change in behavior occur, and work by Steinaker and Bell (1979). Gestalt theory views learning in context and as encouraged through simultaneous mutual interaction, thereby allowing students to develop insight, a basic sense of and feeling for care (Bigge, 1982). Five dimensions of the care learning process have been identified and will be examined.

Five Dimensions of the Learning Process

1. *Focused deliberation.* This process encourages conscious thinking about care and professional caring. The learner should experience a heightened cognitive awareness of care. It has been documented by Leininger and substantiated by Williams (1988) that 86% of entering nursing students verbalize altruistic and humanitarian values as

the primary reasons they enter nursing. Hence, reflection on own past experiences and observation of care will be accentuated.

Each student is asked to reflect on one's experiences as a recipient of care and agent of caring. Discussion will focus on generic care and the meaning of caring to the individual. Clinical field experience begins with student observation of caring in a variety of situations. Parallel observation experiences of generic care, professional care, and professional nurse care are planned. Faculty-led discussion encourages comparison and contrast of care across levels (see Table 1). Discussion should conclude by focusing on the knowledge and clinical skill that demonstrated professional nurse caring. What does knowledge mean in each situation? What specific actions demonstrated caring? Were uncaring behaviors identified? How did clients react to uncaring behaviors? These experiences also demonstrate the contextual nature of nurse caring.

2. *Discovery of care in the clinical context.* These processes aid the student's exploration and revelation of professional nurse caring. Learning experiences take place in actual clinical areas. Constructs of care (Leininger, 1981b) should be integrated into all basic skills that are taught. Curricula in which communication skills and physical assessment are the first nursing skills taught can use presence and touch, as construct of care, to enhance understanding of these skills.

To emphasize to the student and the client that caring is primary to the student's responsibility, the introduction of the student to the prospective client is "I am here to care for you today." "My name is

Table 1
Observations of Care and Caring

Generic Care	Professional Care	Professional Nurse Care
1. Day care center	Kindergarten class	School nurse
2. Homeless mission	Social worker	Public health nurse
3. Family in surgical waiting room	Liaison minister in surgical waiting room	Perioperative admission nurse
4. Lay self-help group	Social worker lead group	Nurse-led lamaze class

Note: Each individual student should have experiences across columns so comparisons can be made in similar situations.

_____ and I am a student nurse." During the practice of communication techniques and interviewing, the topic is the client's perception of caring and caring activities. Beginning students will find this approach more consistent with a nursing perspective than the traditional approach of past illness or family history.

Each student should interview two patients and one nurse from the same clinical field about perceptions of care. Knowledge of cultural and gender differences in caring can be gained by selecting a variety of clients for each student. Reading assignments are selected from English, Australian, and Canadian nursing journals to facilitate the integration of cultural aspects of care (Griffin, 1983; Jones, 1983; Kershaw, 1987; Van Hooft, 1987). These activities will guide the student in the examination of caring from a nursing and client viewpoint.

3. *Confirmation of caring.* Emphasis in this dimension is on clinical field experiences in specific practice settings. Knowledge and technical skill as primary to caring are the focus. Skill learning and theory learning are viewed as the same and seen as occurring in context (Schon, 1987). Application of the concept of care to the basic techniques and technologies of nursing aids the beginning student in realizing that the essential ingredient in professional nursing is care. The manner in which the nurse touches and carries out the procedure connotes the message: "I care." "I respect your dignity and worth" (Reilly & Oermann, 1985, p. 238).

All technical skills are introduced as having a biophysical, affective, and cultural component. In those areas in which information is available about the client's perception of nursing techniques that data is introduced first. Sensory information, information giving, mouth care, and back rubs are examples (Alvino, 1986; Gries & Fernsler, 1988; Johnson, Fuller, Endress, & Rice, 1978; Longworth, 1982; Speedier, 1983). Care constructs such as support, surveillance, and monitoring can be used to structure explanations for specific interventions. Care research is used to document that care is scientific (Brown, 1986; Field, 1984; Swanson-Kauffman, 1986; Ray, 1984). The student should begin to see patterns of caring within nurse-client interactions. Capacity to engage in professional caring behaviors should show beginning evidence.

4. *Transferability of caring.* These types of experiences afford the student the opportunity to use previously learned information in another situation. Orientation to new clinical units is focused on the

student observing and listening to clients' beliefs of care and caring. These findings will be compared and contrasted to past experiences with other clients. Research by Gardener and Wheeler (1981) and Larson (1986, 1987) can be used to reinforce the contextual nature of care.

An experiential diary should be kept in which the student records specific caring activities used. Each activity is then classified according to a list of caring constructs. As caring activities or skills are complied under caring constructs, faculty should assist the student in formulating and modifying professional care actions in new situations. The work of Riemen (1986) on caring and noncaring behaviors is introduced to explore noncaring activities.

Use of cultural data is fostered by asking each student to read an article from a non-English professional journal that has been translated by a member of the foreign language department. Students are encouraged to confirm their understanding with clients from those cultural areas. Examples should be pertinent to the culture of the clients in the immediate population.

5. *Insight Dissemination.* These experiences provide the student the opportunity to apply past information in such a manner that it indicates internal and external knowledge of the professional caring experience. Benner and Wrubel (1989) discussed this as body and mind coming together in a way of knowing. Students are not expected to be "expert practitioners" but they should begin to see relationships that constitute a caring practice as an entity as opposed to discrete actions.

Instead of the traditional care plan, clinical preparation answers the questions "What do I need to know to care for this client?" and "How will I demonstrate care and caring for this client?" Students are encouraged to ask clients to identify strengths and limitations of the care the student gave. A portion of clinical conference time is used for each student to present a conference to peers on how caring was incorporated into a specific nursing skill. And, most important, feedback from clients indicates that clients felt cared for when the student was present.

Virginia Henderson (1985, p. 2) has stated that this is "an age where the psychosocial aspects of nursing have thrown an eclipse on the physical aspects. . . ." This chapter has demonstrated that the use of professional nurse caring, understood as technical skill and knowledge, embodies both of these aspects of nursing. Curriculum revision and pedagogical caring are not sufficient to communicate the value of care. Professional nurse caring, as an interpersonal experience, can only be learned in the clinical field context.

REFERENCES

Aamodt, A. M. (1984). Themes and issues in conceptualizing care. In M. M. Leininger (Ed.), *Care: The essence of nursing and health* (pp. 75–79). Thorofare, NJ: Slack.

Allanach, E. J., & Golden, B. M. (1988). Patients' expectations and values clarification: A service audit. *Nursing Administration Quarterly, 12*(3), 17–22.

Alvino, D. (1986). A caring concept: Providing information to make decisions. *Topics in Clinical Nursing, 8*(2), 70–76.

Benner, P., & Wrubel, J. (1989). *The primacy of caring: Stress and coping in health and illness.* Menlo Park, CA: Addison-Wesley.

Bigge, M. L. (1982). *Learning theories for teachers* (4th ed.). New York: Harper & Row.

Bowman, L. (1988). A phenomenological analysis of the experience of being caring in a nurse-client interaction. *Dissertation Abstracts International, 49,* 73-B-74-B. (University Microfilms No. DA8800194)

Brown, L. (1986). The experience of care: patient perspectives. *Topics in Clinical Nursing, 8*(2), 56–62.

Crisci, P. E. (October 1981). Quest: Helping students learn caring and responsibility. *Phi Delta Kappan,* pp. 131–133.

Cronin, S. N., & Harrison, B. (1988). Importance of nurse caring behaviors as perceived by patients after myocardial infarction. *Heart & Lung, 17,* 374–380.

Fantini, M. D. (November 1980). Disciplined caring. *Phi Delta Kappan,* pp. 182–184.

Field, P. (1984). Client care-seeking behaviors and nursing care. In M. M. Leininger (Ed.), *Care: The essence of nursing and health* (pp. 249–262). Thorofare, NJ: Slack.

Gardner, K. G., & Wheeler, E. (1981). In M. M. Leininger (Ed.), *Caring: An essential human need* (pp. 109–113). Thorofare, NJ: Slack.

Gries, M. L., & Fernsler, J. (1988). Patient perception of the ventilation experience. *Focus on Critical Care, 15*(2), 52–59.

Griffin, A. P. (1983). A philosophical analysis of caring in nursing. *Journal of Advanced Nursing, 8,* 289–295.

Henderson, V. (1985). The essence of nursing in high technology. *Nursing Administration Quarterly, 9*(4), 1–9.

Henry, M. (1975). Nurse behaviors perceived by patients as indicators of caring. *Dissertation Abstracts International, 36,* 652B. (University Microfilms No. 75-16,229)

Hergenhahn, B. R. (1982). *An introduction to theories of learning* (2d ed.). Englewood Cliffs, NJ: Prentice-Hall.

Hult, R. E. (1980). On pedagogical caring. *Educational Theory, 29,* 237–243.

Johnson, J. E., Fuller, S. S., Endress, M. P., & Rice, V. S. (1978). Altering patient's responses to surgery: An extension and replication. *Research in Nursing and Health, 1,* 111–121.

Jones, I. (1983). From a consumer's point of view . . . reactions of one patient to the care he received, *Nursing Times, 79*(31), 31.

Kershaw, B. (1987). Education for care. *Senior Nurse, 6*(6), 28–29.

Larson, P. J. (1986). Cancer nurses' perceptions of caring. *Cancer Nursing, 9*(2), 86–91.

Larson, P. J. (1987). Comparison of cancer patients' and professional nurses' perceptions of important nurse caring behaviors. *Heart & Lung, 16,* 187–193.

Larson, P. J. (1984). Important nurse caring behaviors perceived by patients with cancer. *Oncology Nurse Forum, 11*(6), 46–50.

Leininger, M. M. (1980). Caring: A central focus of nursing and health care service. *Nursing and Health Care, 1*(3), 135–143, 176.

Leininger, M. M. (1981a). Cross-cultural hypothetical functions of caring and nursing care. In M. M. Leininger (Ed.), *Caring: An essential human need.* (pp. 95–102). Thorofare, NJ: Slack.

Leininger, M. M. (1981b). The phenomenon of caring: Importance, research questions and theoretical considerations. In M. M. Leininger (Ed.), *Caring: An essential human need* (pp. 3–15). Thorofare, NJ: Slack.

Leininger, M. M. (1984). Southern rural black and white American lifeways with focus on care and health promotion. In M. M. Leininger (Ed.), *Care: The essence of nursing and health* (pp. 133–159). Thorofare, NJ: Slack.

Leininger, M. M. (1988). Leininger's theory of nursing: Cultural care diversity and universality. *Nursing Science Quarterly, 1,* 152–160.

Longworth, J. C. D. (1982). Psychophysiological effects of slow stroke back massage in normotensive females. *Advances in Nursing Science, 4*(4), 44–61.

Mayer, D. K. (1986). Patients' and families' perceptions of nurse caring behaviors. *Topics in Clinical Nursing, 8*(2), 63–69.

Mayer, D. K. (1987). Oncology nurses' versus cancer patients' perceptions of nurse caring behaviors: A replication study. *Oncology Nurse Forum, 14*(3), 46–52.

Mayeroff, M. (1971). *On caring.* New York: Harper & Row.

Noddings, N. (1984). *Caring: A feminine approach to ethics and moral education.* Berkeley: University of California Press.

Ray, M. A. (1984). The development of a classification system of institutional caring. In M. M. Leininger (Ed.), *Care: The essence of nursing and health* (pp. 95–112). Thorofare, NJ: Slack.

Reilly, D. E., & Oermann, M. H. (1985). *The clinical field: Its use in nursing education.* Norwalk, CT: Appleton-Century-Crofts.

Riemen, D. J. (1986). Noncaring and caring in the clinical setting: Patients' descriptions. *Topics in Clinical Nursing, 8*(2), 30–36.

Schon, D. S. (1987). *Educating the reflective practitioner.* San Francisco: Jossey-Bass.

Servellen, G. van. (1988). Nurses' perceptions of individualized care in nursing practice. *Western Journal of Nursing Research, 10,* 291–306.

Speedier, G. (1983). Nursology of mouth care: Preventing, comforting and seeking activities related to nursing care. *Journal of Advanced Nursing, 8,* 33–40.

Steinaker, N. B., & Bell, M. R. (1979). *The experiential taxonomy: A new approach to teaching and learning.* New York: Harper.

Swanson-Kauffman, D. M. (1986). Caring in the instance of an expected early pregnancy loss. *Topics in Clinical Nursing, 8*(2), 37–46.

Van Hooft, S. (1987). Caring and professional commitment. *Australian Journal of Advanced Nursing, 4*(4), 29–38.

Watson, J. (1988). *Nursing: Human science and human care. A theory of nursing.* New York: National League for Nursing.

Watson, J., Burckhardt, C., Brown, L., Bloch, D., & Hester, N. (1979). A model of caring: An alternative health care model for nursing research and practice. *Clinical and Scientific Sessions.* Kansas City, MO: American Nurses' Association.

Weiss, C. J. (1984). Gender-related perceptions of caring in the nurse-patient relationship. In M. M. Leininger (Ed.), *Care: The essence of nursing and health* (pp. 161–181). Thorofare, NJ: Slack.

Williams, R. P. (1988). College freshmen aspiring to nursing careers: Trends from the 1960s to the 1980s. *Western Journal of Nursing Research, 10*(1), 94–97.

Wilson, P. A. (1986). Informal care and social support: An agenda for the future. *British Journal of Social Work, 16,* 173–179.

Wolf, Z. R. (1986). The caring concept and nurse-identified caring behaviors. *Topics in Clinical Nursing, 8*(2), 84–93.

13

Creative Strategies for Teaching Care

Rauda Gelazis

Care should be taught, within the broadest possible perspective using a variety of creative strategies applicable, on all levels of nursing education. Since cultural care is the broadest context within which to study care, I have based the teaching of care on the Leininger theory and model of nursing (Leininger, 1985, 1988, 1989). Every person, including teacher and student, is unique but each one lives in a context of a particular culture. Thus the individual is linked to groups and culture by way of the family and kinship group. Diversity and uniqueness, when understood from an emic (insider's) perspective (Leininger, 1985, 1988; Luna & Cameron, 1989), can provide a framework for understanding care.

Nurse educators need to encourage and promote all ways of knowing to empower future nurses to be able to respond as complete human beings in caring ways to their clients (Stein, 1986). In recent years, nurse scholars are beginning to realize that a narrow way of thinking is detrimental to nursing (Carper, 1978). More and more nurse authors are discussing the importance of expanding our knowledge and in turn our ways of teaching at all levels of nursing education (Dzurec, 1989).

Creativity has been an object of study in a variety of fields from psychology to psychophysiology (Bogen & Bogen, 1988). Nursing, however, has only recently shown interest in creativity. If we are to continue to develop as a discipline, we must pay more attention to creativity. Nurse educators need to foster the creative process rather than discourage it (Bush, 1988). Through the creative process new and workable approaches to unsolved problems or previously unrecognized solutions or opportunities are recognized. The solution usually seems to appear somewhat suddenly as a whole framework or approach and details are filled in later.

Some authors have pointed out that creativity seems to occur in stages (Krystal, 1988). Initially there is a dormant stage when nothing seems to occur. The person puts away the question or problem for a time, then all of a sudden comes up with a new solution or approach (Zdanek, 1988). In this manner, the left hemisphere of the brain is first used to logically approach the problem, then in the dormant phase, the right hemisphere has a chance to operate in a different manner. Recently, the role of the corpus callosum in its central location between the two hemispheres has been identified as central to the creative process for creativity depends to some extent on transcallosal interhemispheric exchange (Bogen & Bogen, 1988). In the past, nursing education has focused on left-brain types of learning—that is, logical processes in thought and expression. I contend that today nurse educators must include a variety of approaches to teaching to educate the full person.

Particularly because care has many aspects, it should be taught using a variety of creative teaching strategies. I will propose several creative strategies for teaching care to empower nurses and student nurses to truly respond to clients in caring ways congruent with their cultures. These strategies include use of poetry, use of humor, promotion of a sense of wonder, work with other cultural groups (such as the homeless), awareness of popular culture, and use of arts as drama.

USE OF POETRY

In the teaching of care for the mentally ill I use the creative strategy of poetry. Part of the goal in teaching psychiatric mental health nursing is to increase students' sensitivity to clients and their families and to their own reactions to the needs and feelings of mentally ill clients. Such sensitivity must be opened in the relatively short time of seven weeks. Initially I give examples of poems expressing needs of patients such as the need to be listened to and empathized with (Gelazis, 1988). Therefore, poems are discussed in clinical conference and in theory classes in relation to clients. Poems are also being used in various settings (Taft, 1989). At the end of the rotation in psychiatric mental health nursing, students are given the option to write a poem about their experiences. Students are told that they can use any poetic form and can choose as subject any aspect of their experiences, such as their own feelings, emotions, perceptions about themselves, their clients, or the experience as a whole. Keeping the assignments broad and open allows for creativity of approach as does the poetic format. Students who are too threatened by such an assignment, who have said "I can't write a poem!" can opt for a more traditional assignment. When students share their poems in conference, all are usually amazed at the variety of topics, forms of expression, and depth of insight expressed.

In planning this assignment for senior nursing students I believe that I provide an opportunity for synthesis of learning to occur. Students can put together in one assignment aspects that they learned in past liberal arts courses such as psychology, cultural anthropology, or literature with their nursing experience. Care and other aspects of their nursing experience can then be given an expression in a poetic form. Here teaching and learning occur in a holistic manner—that is, right and left brain activity occur in the process of creating a poem.

Feelings and emotions are an important part of life. In the past, a nurse was taught about feelings regarding her patient, but her own reactions were to be "controlled" or even ignored in order to be "objective" about patients. Today we recognize that nurses do have feelings. We need to teach students to recognize, clearly identify, and then act on these feelings in appropriate ways. We need to be aware of and use our emotional selves, our spiritual selves, and our social and cultural selves for the well-being of our clients and families. We also need to be aware of these aspects within a wider context of culture and world. When students' poems are discussed by teacher and students, the meaning and cultural context for the student and the client need to be incorporated. Symbols used in the poem and their cultural meanings can be discussed as well. In this way care can be incorporated in view of a broader context.

Several examples illustrate newly found perceptions in students. "thoughts on a gelid morning" by Stephanie Bower (see poem 1) shows extreme sensitivity and expresses a synthesis of several perspectives important to a nurse. This student speaks of an "inner care" and implies the spirituality that is important to nurses. Her own questions and issues are raised by her culture in which the demanding roles of an adult, a wife and mother, must be balanced in pursuing her dream of becoming a nurse. This poem reminds me of the tacit knowing that we have and use, particularly in nursing (Polanyi, 1966). This form of knowing is difficult to express and can't really be measured. I believe it is illustrated in this student's sensitivity.

In the next student poem, Elke Vogt expresses a deep empathy. Empathy has been described as a part of caring (Leininger, 1988). Neurophysiologists and biologists have studied the nature of empathy, noting that during the evolution of primate central nervous systems, organization of neural activity was shaped by the need for rapid and accurate evaluation of the motivations of others—empathy (Horton, 1988). Thus, in a sense, our survival as a human race has depended on our ability to empathize. Poem 2 shows empathy; in fact it is written from the client's viewpoint describing a boy who recovers his sense of self-worth through a riding program. On his horse, he can be tall, on eye level with others in his environment.

In poem 3, student Carol Manuel describes the essence of nursing—caring. In "I Care . . . Therefore I Am a Nurse" she points out how essential care is in the nurse. It is the very life of nursing. This poem gets to the case of what nursing is about.

Another part of this assignment is that once the poems are written and discussed, some are selected to be submitted to nursing journals. In this manner the importance of sharing through publication is emphasized. Also the process of how to have one's written work published becomes a real aspect of students' learning experiences.

POEM 1
Stephanie Bower

thoughts on a gelid morning

i see myself reflected in the car window, weary, angry with myself at the idea of failing my family. am i neglecting them because i selfishly want to do what i feel called to do? if i have failed them; then, everything i've done is of no worth.

again, sipping coffee, i see myself; but, this time my reflection is not in the window. it appears in the faces of those around me who are also tired, worn, sick of the struggle of life. WAIT. i see something more in these faces. i behold vulnerability, and this state cradles a pride, a dignity, a respect that is striking. this is the essence of us. for withinside this openness we are able to search deep within our souls and call upon a strength much greater outside ourselves. it is in this place where we meet ourselves and our creator and question life and its purpose.

it is here, the locus of our being, where we truly begin to feel, regenerate, and restore our sight and perchance, connect with the universe. to become a part of all that is, was, and will be. in each of us this place resides. once we've been there our lives are changed forever.

perceiving ourselves and others with this restored sight, we can no longer experience others as different, but become as one; therefore, seeing our own reflection in all of man and nature. realizing this, we can no longer crush the other. this spiritual resurrection demands that we uphold ourselves and others with dignity and respect.

this place dubbed vulnerability instills in us a reverence, and we are to move and breathe within this proclamation.

POEM 2
Elke Vogt

There was a time, long past, my heart was free
to ride the waves and run in the fields and be
whatever fantastic thing I wanted to be.
An accident, a crashing fall,
a cruel attack, ended it all.
And I am left alone to sit and stare
and watch the world go by from my metal chair,
lost in the dark abyss of deep despair.
They put me on a horse one day
to help and pass the time away.
Sitting tall on his back I could meet others face to face
for they'd look at me and see ME, not my wheelchair and brace.
He changed my world, my horse, my gentle friend.
He helped me to take up the reins of life again.

POEM 3
Carol Manuel

I Care . . . Therefore I Am a Nurse

I care
   Therefore I am a Nurse
I listen
   Therefore I am attentive to your needs

I feel
  Therefore I am aware of your presence
I understand
  Therefore I perceive the meaning of you
I respect
  Therefore I admire you as a person and will not judge you
I enable
  Therefore I give back to you authority over your life
I comfort
  Therefore I have compassion for you
I reason
  Therefore I think about, understand and conclude about you
I help
  Therefore if you need to, you can rely on me
I love
  Therefore your life is important to me
I nurture
  Therefore I will nourish and rear you
I motivate
  Therefore I encourage you to be independent
I trust
  Therefore I initiate you to be confident and self reliant
I encourage
  Therefore I give you hope and confidence
I advocate
  Therefore I will plead on your behalf, and inform you of your rights
I advise
  Therefore I give advice, recommend, inform and notify you
I exist . . .
  Therefore you have a chance

USE OF HUMOR

A second creative strategy for the teaching of care involves humor.
Creative traits in people have been linked with a sense of humor
(Goldstein & McGhee, 1972). Humor can be an important part of caring for clients, caring for other nurses, and caring for ourselves. Humor
can be taught to all levels of nurses and nursing students. However,
there may be considerable "unlearning" that needs to be done by some.
If we look at the culture of nursing historically, we can see that for the
most part, nurses have been taught and socialized to maintain a serious
demeanor while caring for clients. Many nurses may remember being

reprimanded by head nurses or nursing instructors for too much joking and laughter or not being serious enough.

Of course, one may wonder what to do with a humorless student or nurse. The answer is that there is a core in each person that was once a child with spontaneity, lightheartedness, and an ability to play (all needed to some degree for humor to occur). This sensitivity for humor or to life's lighter side can be gradually increased in each nurse or student.

A first step that may be important to the teaching of humor is to help students and nurses to become aware of the taboos against humor that we have imposed on ourselves or have had imposed from others. An inventory of such taboos may be useful. This inventory can be made by asking others or oneself to complete the following sentence with ten or more reasons: "Humor and playfulness are not very 'adult' or 'professional' because. . . ." Once people answer these for themselves, a discussion about the taboos can follow to determine how much these are believed and adhered to in nurse-client interactions.

Once we become aware of the level of humor and lightheartedness in our lives, we can decide how they can be increased. Humor calls for genuineness and the ability to be yourself without hiding behind roles.

Some examples of teaching and learning activities for incorporating humor include the following:

1. Acting as a role model for humor and care. Our students learn a great deal from us by emulating our behaviors. Therefore, if we can use humor in caring ways to clients, students, other nurses, and professionals, our students will have role models to follow.

2. Keeping a humor diary. This involves writing down a note or two in a specific place, when something humorous happens. At the end of the day, one may write the funniest thing that happened or note a joke that was well received by a client or a student. Very frequently, if certain kinds of jokes or humor don't go over well, the reason may be because it was not culturally congruent with the client or family. For example, a New England joke may fall flat when told to persons from the midwest or other parts of the country.

3. Telling short humorous stories or jokes. These can be told and exchanged, as well as critiqued, in small group settings and discussions. An instructor that I had in graduate school assigned the class to have a joke to tell the next class day. During the joke time, the stories or jokes were shared. Usually the teacher had the joke time when

energy and interest waned. The humor acted as a natural form of reenergizing and created group interest and energy.

4. Collecting and incorporating cartoons into class presentations or discussions. Many "Peanuts" cartoons have illustrated a point without many words, but the point is well noted and remembered. For example, students or instructors can discuss transcultural nursing with the help of well-known cartoon characters such as Garfield.

These are just a few of the ways that humor can become a part of our teaching as well as our way of interacting with clients and students. Humor, when used appropriately in culturally congruent ways, can become a creative strategy for teaching care. For through humor we can care for ourselves as well as clients and other nurses or health care providers.

ENCOURAGING A SENSE OF WONDER

Another creative strategy for teaching care is encouraging a sense of wonder about life and human beings, as well as our world in our students. Encouraging a sense of wonder helps students remain open to new knowledge. Undergraduate nursing students frequently take courses such as cultural anthropology, but may not be able to relate such courses to themselves or to clients. For example, students have said, "We just learned about a few extinct tribes" and dismiss what they learned about culture. The instructor needs to help students learn about themselves and their own cultural backgrounds. Students can be taught how to do a mini-ethnonursing study using their own families as informants. By researching personal roots, cultural patterns, values, and beliefs can be shared with classmates. Such a strategy can increase an awareness of the cultural diversity in students. From such a beginning can come an appreciation of how cultural care can be appropriately given to clients from various cultures.

WORK WITH THE HOMELESS

Students can be helped to experience caring for a population such as the homeless to learn how to appreciate and care for a diverse population of clients. For example, students can be assigned to an emergency room or psychiatric emergency room where homeless clients may have contact with the health care system. One student who was given such an opportunity also rode in a police car when police took a homeless client to a shelter in midwinter. This experience was an eye-opener to the student. She had had contact with minority cultures, but found herself shocked by the way that the homeless person was treated. She noted that he was given no choice about going to a shelter by the police. The person was obviously mentally ill, but was not attended to. The many problems and issues related to this one visit were part of the discussion with students following this experience. Ways of caring for this population were discussed.

CARE VIA POPULAR CULTURE

Students in all levels of nursing education programs frequently have a narrow focus of education. Many students are so intent on learning their profession that they lose touch with current events. One strategy for helping students open to broad knowledge is to assign them to read a book from the best-seller list. Students can then report and share what they learned. Not only is the book reported on, but also the background of the book and author as well as the field knowledge. The Leininger Sunrise model can be a way of understanding the various aspects that students identify. For example, if the book is about politics or economics, that part of the model can be explained by the student. In this manner all parts of the sunrise can be discussed by the students.

CARE THROUGH THE ARTS

Drama can be used to illustrate culturally congruent care. Students can select a particular culture during a semester, study this culture, and then write a short play to demonstrate their knowledge of the culture and care appropriate to clients of this culture. Another group of students may select to illustrate their culture through painting, collage, or graphic art. In this manner various cultures would be explored by students by means of different art forms. Another way to use the arts would be to attend a play together and later discuss what was learned. For example, recently in our area, there was a play about a group home dealing with their problems. This would be an excellent way to discuss some of the issues that mentally ill clients face at discharge. The political and health care systems can also be part of the discussion of such a play.

The theoretical underpinnings for these creative strategies can be found in Leininger (1985), Watson (1979), and others. The limit and scope of this presentation prevent developing the theory here, but this is a very important part of the above creative strategies for teaching care. Without understanding the overall meaning that a theory can give to any single teaching strategy, no matter how successful or creative, the student is left at a practice level of his or her discipline. The theoretical underpinnings, when understood in light of the philosophy of nursing being presented, help to elevate both student and teacher to higher and higher levels of meaning and abstraction. In this manner, our discipline is thereby developed. Such creative approaches to teaching care to students and to broadening their knowledge need to be further developed and results studied.

CONCLUSION

I would like to challenge you to be as creative as possible in teaching care, for I believe that each of us is a potential teacher of care. Cultural care, as I have illustrated here, can be a framework for such activity.

REFERENCES

Bogen, J. E., & Bogen, G. M. (1986). Creativity and the corpus callosum. *Psychiatric Clinics of North America, 11*(3), 293–301.

Bush, H. A. (1988). The caring teacher in nursing. In M. M. Leininger (Ed.), *Care: Discovery and Uses in Clinical and Community Nursing.* Detroit: Wayne State University Press. 11–28.

Carper, B. A. (1978). Fundamental patterns of knowing in nursing. *Advances in Nursing Science, 1*(1), 13–23.

Dzurec, L. C. (1989). The necessity for and evolution of multiple paradigms for nursing research: A poststructualist perspective. *Advances in Nursing Science, 11*(4), 69–77.

Horton, P. C. (1988). Positive emotions and the right parietal cortex. *Psychiatric Clinics of North America, 11*(3), 1461–1474.

Gelazis, R. (1988). Empathy. *Nursing Forum, 2,* 55.

Goldstein, J. H., & McGhee, P. E. (1972). *The psychology of humor: Theoretical perspectives and empirical issues.* New York: Academic Press.

Krystal, H. (1988). On some roots of creativity. *Psychiatric Clinics of North America, 11*(3), 475–491.

Leininger, M. M (1985). Transcultural care diversity and universality: A theory of nursing. *Nursing and Health Care, 4,* 209–212.

Leininger, M. M. (1988). Leininger's theory of nursing: Cultural care diversity and universality. *Nursing Science Quarterly, 1*(4), 152–160.

Leininger, M. M. (1989). History, issues, and trends in the discovery and uses of care in nursing. In M. M. Leininger (Ed.), *Care: Discovery and Uses in Clinical and Community Nursing.* Detroit: Wayne State University Press, 11–28.

Luna, L., & Cameron, C. (1989). *Leininger's transcultural nursing.* In J. J. Fitzpatrick & A. L. Whall (Eds.), *Conceptual Models of Nursing* (2 ed.), 227–239.

Polanyi, M. (1966). *The tacit dimension.* New York: Anchor Press, p. 4.

Sarter, B. (1988). Philosophical sources of nursing theory. *Nursing Science Quarterly, 1*(2), 52–59.

Stein, A. P. (1986). Teaching nurses to care. *Nurse Educator, 11*(6), 4.

Taft, L. B. (1989). Remembering and sharing through poetry writing. *Nurse Educator, 14*(1), 37–38.

Watson, J. (1985). *Nursing: Human science and human care. A theory of nursing.* Norwalk, CT: Appleton-Century-Crofts.

Watson, J. (1979). *Nursing: The philosophy and science of caring.* Boston: Little, Brown.

Zdanek, M. (1988). Right-brain techniques: A catalyst for creative thinking and internal focusing. *Psychiatric Clinics of North America, 11*(3), 427–446.

14

Teaching Care as the Essence of Nursing Administration

Christina L. S. Evans

The directors of nursing departments within health care settings are, generally, nurses. However, not all directors of nursing demonstrate professional nursing concerns as they fulfill the expectations of their position. I have often observed that directors demonstrate managerial concerns similar to those of their superiors—the hospital administrators and/or medical staff. Financial concerns become the priority rather than patient concerns. However, other directors of nursing do demonstrate professional nursing concerns. Patients are their priority focus, not the meeting of budgetary constraints. What makes the difference between these two groups of nurses? Why does one group seemingly care, and one group apparently not care?

I propose that there are two groups of nurses in management: nurse-managers and managers with nursing backgrounds. Nurse-managers demonstrate professional nursing concerns, while managers with nursing backgrounds demonstrate managerial concerns. I further propose that the primary difference between the two groups is the ability of a nurse-manager to value and care for a nursing department as a client.

In this chapter, I propose that care is the essence of nursing management and should be incorporated into nursing management curriculum. First, I present the potential benefits of valuing care by nurse-managers in contrast to the potential results when care is not valued. Next, techniques for incorporating care into nursing management-curriculum will be developed. Finally, directions for research will be presented.

WHY NURSE-MANAGERS SHOULD CARE

I believe that nurse-managers are practicing nursing. They do not relinquish the ability to deliver care when they become nurse-managers; they change their client focus. As a staff nurse, the individual is the focus of care—the client. A staff nurse provides care to an individual. When a staff nurse becomes a nurse-manager, a nursing department is the focus of care—a nurse-manager's client. A nurse-manager provides care to a nursing department as his or her client.

Leininger (1986, 1989) stated that "care is the essence of nursing" (p. 2). Since I propose that nurse-managers continue to practice nursing but with a different client focus, then nurse-managers need to provide professional care to their client (the nursing department). According to Leininger (1981b), professional care "embodies the cognitive and deliberate goals, processes, and acts of professional persons or groups providing assistance to others, and expressing attitudes and actions of concerns for them, in order to support their well-being, alleviate undue discomforts, and meet obvious or anticipated needs" (p. 46). Consistent with the care perspective, needs and well-being are defined from the nursing department's perspective, not from the perspective of the nurse-manager. It is the nurse-manager's responsibility to care for and support the nursing department's achievement of well-being as the essence of nursing management.

Thompson (1986) identified behaviors of nurse-managers who provide care to a nursing department. Characteristics of the caring nurse-manager include an honest, fair, and consistent approach when interacting with the nursing department and its members. The nurse-manager demonstrates care by listening emphatically to departmental members and being attuned to the concerns of the nursing staff. In assisting, supporting, and facilitating the activities and efforts of the nursing department and its members, the nurse-manager provides care to the department and supports the department's achievement of well-being.

A CHOICE FOR NURSE-MANAGERS

Nurses in managerial positions can decide whether to value or to discount care both in terms of their interactions with their client (nursing department) and interactions of individual nurses with their individual patients. As recently as 1986, Leininger stated that "care is not that explicit and sometimes not even identified in . . . service institutions" (p. 4). Many nurses in managerial positions apparently have not chosen to value care, and this has consequences for the nursing management of departments.

Impact of Discounting Care

Managers with nursing background may choose to discount care to resolve the moral conflict that results from the contrasting values of the dominant and subordinate cultures (cure versus care) within health care settings. By discounting care, they attempt to deny its existence and more comfortably identify with the dominant values. However, as a result of this process, the manager with nursing background risks presenting an image of a manager and no longer being recognized or valued as a nurse.

The practice environment becomes focused on values espoused by hospital administration. Efficiency and cost containment become the dominant action modes, and there is little time provided to give care to patients. Marz (1986) identified that caring can be impaired or reinforced by the environment. If the practice environment discounts care, the delivery of care to patients will be impaired or, possibly, absent from the health care setting.

The discounting of care may result in intensifying the moral conflict (regarding the value of care) experienced by the department as a whole. An associated emphasis on the technical (medical) aspect of nursing creates confusion as to whether care is of any value to nursing. This continuing conflict can also result in competition and divisiveness within the department (Roberts, 1983).

The increase in conflict may also result in an increased dissatisfaction among department members. The department is being told to devalue what the educational process indicated was important. With increased dissatisfaction may come increased burnout among department members. In turn, increased burnout may result in increased turnover in the department.

Nurses who do not value care also create a vulnerable situation for individual patients (Ray, 1981a). The individual patient may receive a minimal amount, or a poor quality, of care. The health of the individual patient will not be enhanced, and the consequences of this may include more time in the health care setting, increased complications, and a greater recidivism.

By discounting care, the manager with a nursing background has not supported his or her client (nursing department) to achieve well-being. To the contrary, this manager has facilitated the development of a lower level of functioning by the client (delivery of less quality care to individual patients). This behavior could be perceived to contribute to the development of client (departmental) illness—dissatisfaction, job incongruencies, increased turnover.

Impact of Valuing Care

Buerhaus (1986), Leininger (1981b, 1986), and Ray (1987) have identified that it is important for care to be valued within health care settings. Leininger (1986) stated that the "caring role . . . must be openly recognized, legitimized, and facilitated in places where cultural taboos and myths have limited [its] 'optional' functioning" (pp. 5–6). Leininger further identified that "most people come to the hospital to receive care . . . what people want and need most from nurses has been and still remains quality humanized care" (p. 9).

Departmental Impact. Four major areas will be affected by the nurse-manager's decision to value and promote care: the nursing department, the patient, the hospital, and the nurse-manager.

For the nurse-manager to provide care to his or her client (the nursing department), care must be emphasized and integrated throughout departmental activities. The orientation of new nursing staff should incorporate the concept of caring and the care constructs. This process will assure that new employees will recognize and value the importance of care. The nursing department should also evaluate its ability to provide care. Hence, job descriptions and their associated performance evaluations should emphasize care as a major component. Care should also be incorporated into the acuity or patient classification system used by the department to ensure that the nurses have time to care for individual patients.

In addition, the nurse-manager should ensure that rewards are associated with the provision of care by nurses. These rewards can either be financial (Leininger, 1986) or intrinsic (rewards that a nurse receives from the provision of care) (Ray, 1981a). Ray hypothesized that nurses who provide care to patients should experience increased self-esteem, increased motivation, and increased job satisfaction. In addition, I propose that turnover will decrease and retention increase as a result of the nurses' increased satisfaction with their work environment.

Impact on Individual Clients. The individual clients receiving care from nurses will also benefit from care being valued within a nursing department. Bush and Kjervik (1979) state that "better" nursing is provided by nurses with positive self-images. Just as the department benefits, nurses will also experience increased self-esteem when working within a nursing department that values care (Ray, 1981a). Hence, it can be proposed that individual clients will receive improved nursing in health care settings where care is valued. Ray further proposes that patients will also experience a decreased length of stay and require fewer readmissions.

Impact on the Health Care Setting. The health care setting, generally the hospital, will also benefit from the nurse-manager's decision to value and promote care to his or her client. As early as 1981(b), Ray stated that "hospital caring was now a 'big business' and financial administrators often referred to caring as a function of the hospital's economic health" (p. 109). With the increasing emphasis on competition and cost containment within the health care environment, Buerhaus (1986) proposed that "most hospitals will promote 'high quality patient care' as one of their chief products" (p. 16). If a nurse-manager can help his or her department achieve well-being—which includes, as one component, the effective delivery of care to all individual clients—the hospital will benefit from an improved public image and a probable associated increase in market share.

Impact on the Nurse-Manager. The nurse-manager may possibly experience negative outcomes from the decision to value and promote care to his or her client (nursing department). The existence and extent of the negative outcomes depend on the nurse-manager's ability to change values within the culture of the health care setting. The nurse-manager who intends to value and promote care must serve as a change agent to assure that the health care setting culture values care as defined by his or her client (nursing department). The ability of the nurse-manager to succeed in this process depends on his or her relationship with superiors and ability to use the health care setting's culture and language to facilitate change. By being able to communicate the benefits to the health care setting that result from valuing care, the nurse-manager will facilitate the nursing department's progress as it implements strategies to value and promote care (Buerhaus, 1986; Ray, 1987).

Ultimately, the nurse-manager should also experience the intrinsic rewards experienced by all nurses within a department where care is valued: increased self-esteem, increased motivation, and increased job satisfaction (Ray, 1981a). Initially, however, the nurse-manager may experience increased stress and conflict as his or her actions may be perceived to threaten the health care setting culture's power and authority. The policy of "employment at will" (the ability of the nurse-manager's superior to terminate the nurse-manager's employment without due process or cause) indicates that the nurse-manager remains in the position at the discretion of his or her superior. Therefore, it is important for the nurse-manager to utilize the health care setting culture's values when beginning the change process. I expect that, once care is valued and promoted by the nursing department, benefits to the health care setting culture (hospital and physicians) will provide additional support and momentum for continued changes.

CURRICULUM FOR CARING IN NURSING ADMINISTRATION

Davis (1987) stated "the essence of any nursing curriculum should be nursing" (p. 285). And, assuming the essence of nursing is care (Leininger, 1986, p. 2), it logically proceeds that the essence of any nursing curriculum should be care. Hence, nursing management curriculum should also have a care focus.

King and Gerwig (1981) emphasized that curriculum should reflect "what the profession can and should be, rather than merely reflecting current practice" (p. 26). Since it is crucial for both the quality of health care and the retention/recruitment of nurses that nurse-managers practice care, it is imperative that current nursing management curriculum focus on care. This focus will then result in nurse-managers who care for their clients.

Various strategies can be used to incorporate care into nursing management curriculum beginning at undergraduate level coursework. A new curriculum can be instituted which addresses care from the nurse-management perspective or current curriculum focusing on administrative and management theories can integrate care into all aspects of coursework. A caring theory-based nursing management curriculum should address research into nursing management practices and systems of caring and emphasize the relationship between human and system caring approaches and positive departmental and organizational outcomes (Watson, 1988).

Content included in a management administration curriculum focusing on care should include:

1. Care constructs as applied to nursing management.
2. Care theory as applied to nursing management.
3. Development of care skills within nursing management contexts.
4. Changing cultures to value and reward caring behaviors.
5. A practicum.

The practicum would synthesize the student's previously learned knowledge within the context of an actual health care setting. By identifying caring behaviors as they occur during the observational period, the student can serve as an educator to current nursing managers. This identification process will increase the nurse-managers' awareness of the presence or absence of caring behaviors. The impact of valuing care on the delivery of care, the department, and the health care setting can also be discussed.

RESEARCH IMPLICATIONS

My search to understand the different behaviors of nurses in managerial positions has generated many research questions. A few of them include:

• Do nurses in managerial positions care for their nursing departments?
• How do nurse-managers care for nursing departments?
• What is the culture of nursing departments in which care is valued and promoted?
• What is the culture of nursing departments in which care is not valued and promoted?
• What are the departmental outcomes in nursing departments which value care?

These research questions require the use of qualitative research methods for study. The ethnonursing method proposed by Leininger (1985) would be the method of choice for several reasons.

Ethnonursing lends itself to research situations in which very little information exists regarding a particular culture. Very few publications address the concept of the culture of a nursing department as a whole. Much additional work is needed if theories are to be developed to assist nurse-managers to deliver care to their clients (nursing departments).

The need to address the culture of the nursing department as a whole is another reason for the selection of ethnonursing as a methodology. I believe in the importance of viewing the client of a nurse in a holistic fashion, not as an integration of parts. To view the nursing department holistically, a methodology is needed that supports this holistic approach.

Ethnonursing would also be selected as a research methodology as the author would be studying a nursing phenomena. Ethnonursing focuses "on examining selected nursing and ethnographic data that are related to care, health, prevention of illness states, illness, and other nursing care phenomena" (Leininger, 1985, p. 58). The author would be gathering emic data from nurse informants, and ethnonursing is a methodology that "explicate[s] and document[s] specific nursing care data from the . . . nurses, or nursing, or health situations" (1985, p. 38). The purpose of the author's research would be to understand both the culture of a nursing department and the delivery of care by nurse-managers within that culture. This purpose would be consistent with the goal of ethnonursing: to "discover nursing knowledge as known, perceived, and experienced by nurses" (1985, p. 38).

Ethnonursing's focus on emic data is also considered in the selection of this method. It is the beliefs, assumptions, and values within a nursing department that determine its culture. Only the members of that culture can identify this data. By using ethnonursing methodology, the author can begin to understand the nursing department culture from the perspective of the individuals involved.

Finally, ethnonursing would be selected as a research methodology because it facilitates the finding of meaning within context. The ability of the nursing department to attain a state of well-being is dependent on the culture of the overall health care setting in which the department exists. Without the ability to consider this important factor (the larger culture) as it affects the nurse-manager's client (the nursing department), resulting theoretical knowledge would be limited in its application.

SUMMARY

Not all nurses in managerial positions care for their clients (nursing departments). It is imperative that nurses in managerial positions implement strategies that will enable all nurses to value care. By focusing a nursing management curriculum on care, nurse-managers will value care and incorporate care into their nursing departments. "Health care delivery systems of this nation are currently dominated by an industrial management model. . . . Such a model presents serious conflict with a care culture and nursing, having mastered the current management model, must now move to merge it with the essentials of a care culture. Only then will we create new nursing models which will be responsive to the health care needs of the 21st century" (Krauss, 1988, p. 1).

REFERENCES

Buerhaus, P. I. (1986). The economics of care: Challenges and new opportunities for nursing. *Transcultural Nursing, 8*(2), 13–21.

Bush, M. A. & Kjervik, D. K. (1979). The nurse's self-image. In D. K. Kjervik & I. M. Martinson (Eds.), *Women in stress: A nursing perspective* (pp. 46–47). New York: Appleton-Century-Crofts.

Davis, G. C. (1987). Keeping the focus on nursing. *Nursing Outlook, 35*(6), 285–287.

King, V., & Gerwig, N. (1981). *Humanizing nursing education: A confluent approach through group process.* Wakefield, MA: Nursing Resources.

Krauss, J. B. (1988). Creating a new culture of care. *Archives of Psychiatric Nursing, 2*(1), 1–2.

Leininger, M. M. (1981a). Caring: A central focus of nursing and health care services. In M. M. Leininger (Ed.), *Care: The essence of nursing and health* (pp. 45–59). New York: Slack.

Leininger, M. M. (1981b). Caring is nursing: Understanding the meaning, importance, and issues. In M. M. Leininger (Ed.), *Care: The essence of nursing and health* (pp. 83–93). New York: Slack.

Leininger, M. M. (1985). Ethnography and ethnonursing: Models and modes of qualitative data analysis. In M. M. Leininger (Ed.), *Qualitative research methods in nursing* (pp. 33–71). Orlando, FL: Grune & Stratton.

Leininger, M. M. (1986). Care facilitation and resistance factors in the culture of nursing. *Transcultural Nursing, 8*(2), 1–12.

Leininger, M. M. (1989). Cultural care theory and nursing administration. In B. Henry, C. Arndt, M. Di Vincenti, & A. Marriner-Tomey (Eds.), *Dimensions of nursing administration: Theory, research, education, practice* (pp. 19–34). Boston: Blackwell.

Marz, M. S. (1986). Conceptual care model for reducing stress of newly employed nurses. In P. Brenner, C. Boyd, T. C. Thompson, M. S. Marz, P. Buerhaus, & M. M. Leininger, The care symposium: Considerations for nursing administrators (p. 29). *Journal of Nursing Administration, 16*(1), 25–30.

Ray, M. A. (1981a). A philosophical analysis of caring with nursing. In M. M. Leininger (Ed.), *Caring: An essential human need* (pp. 25–36). Thorofare, NJ: Slack.

Ray, M. A. (1981b). The development of a classification system of institutional caring. In M. M. Leininger (Ed.), *Care: The essence of nursing and health* (pp. 95–111). New York: Slack.

Ray, M. A. (1987). Health care economics and human caring in nursing: Why the moral conflict must be resolved. *Family and Community Health, 10*(1), 35–43.

Roberts, S. J. (1983). Oppressed group behavior: Implications for nursing. *Advances in Nursing Science, 5*(7), 21–30.

Thompson, C. (1986). Discovering the meaning and expressions of care by nursing service directors. In P. Brenner, C. Boyd, T. C. Thompson, M. S. Marz, P. Buerhaus, & M. M. Leininger, The care symposium: Considerations for nursing administrators (p. 28). *Journal of Nursing Administration, 16*(1), 25–30.

Watson, J. (1988). Human caring as moral context for nursing education. *Nursing & Health Care, 9*(1), 423–425.

15

Virtue, Ethics, and Care: Developing the Personal Dimension of Caring in Nursing Education

Mark Klimek

A prevalent theme in current literature on the state of the art in nursing is the proposition that the profession must focus upon care and caring. Leininger (1988) identifies care as the essence and "central, unifying, dominant domain" (p. 3) of nursing. Gaut (1988) summarizes the literature by describing care as a traditional value in nursing and caring as a fundamental and useful component of nursing.

Another common idea expressed by nurse leaders is the neglect of the moral foundation of nursing. Watson (1988) claims that nursing education is conducted in an atmosphere that often ignores the philosophical and moral context of nursing activity. Of particular concern to Watson is the separation of education in health and human caring from a moral and philosophical base. Such concern is not unique to nursing. The same theme is echoed in journals of business, education, and medicine.

Ethicist Howard A. Slaate (1988) asserts that the most crucial challenge for the present generation of Americans is a recovery of moral principles. This challenge must be accepted by nursing educators. This chapter suggests a strategy to address the challenge. It investigates the

177

validity of the concept of virtue in nursing education and examines the contribution of virtue ethics in developing the personal dimension of caring in the professional nurse. Developing a personal virtue of caring based on a well-explicated ethic of care is posited as one potential means to recover the moral foundation of nursing practice.

CARE, CARING, AND VIRTUE

Clarity in definition of terms is essential. The manner in which the terms care, caring, and virtue are conceptualized and defined serves as a basis for discussion of the relationships among them:

> Care—consists of those assistive, supportive or facilitative acts toward, or for another individual or group with evident or anticipated needs, to ameliorate or improve a human condition or lifeway (Leininger, 1988, p. 4).

Care has also been identified as an ethic. As Fry (1988a) affirms, care meets the four requirements for an ethical standard. Care is a paramount value to guide the actions of a nurse. Care is a universal that is appropriate across many contexts and cultures. Care identifies specific behaviors that are considered to characterize excellence. Finally, care is "other-regarding" (p. 48). Care is the central and essential ethic in nursing. The position of this chapter is that nursing ethics is the ethics of care.

Caring is conceptualized as an expression of the nurse. Caring is a human phenomenon with personal and cultural dimensions:

> Caring—is the direct, or indirect, nurturant, skillful activities, processes, and behaviors related to assisting people in such a manner that reflects behavioral attributes which are empathetic, supportive, compassionate, protective, succorant, educational, and others dependent upon the needs, problems, values, and goals of the individual or group being assisted (Leininger, 1988, p. 4).

Brody (1988) states that caring is the focal virtue in nursing. The virtuous nurse demonstrates caring.

Dent discusses virtue as an expression of the whole self (1986). This directly relates virtue to the personal dimension:

> Virtue—is a spontaneous, and consistent aspiration by an individual
> to unequivocally express basic traits of excellent character that fa-
> cilitates action from a moral and philosophical base (Dent, 1986;
> Meilaender, 1984).

Banner (1968) speaks of virtue as the shape or thrust of a person's
character. Expression of virtue does not depend on circumstances, nor
is it conditional (Simon, 1986).

Before moving to the relationship between care, caring, and virtue, it
is important to disclaim a popular view of virtue. Brody (1988), among
others, relates virtue to beneficence and duty. Confusion results when
virtue is based on a sense of duty (Fry, 1988b). Expression of virtue is an
aspiration, not an obligation. Linking virtue with duty is a deontological
notion that makes conscientiousness the supreme human excellence
(Dent, 1984). The moral question for virtue is "What shall I be?" (Walton,
1986), rather than "What does the role demand?"

Care, caring, and virtue are conceptualized to have a distinctive
pattern of relationship. Care, as the ethic of nursing, is the standard to
which professional decisions and actions should be compared. Care is
the standard for doing.

Virtue is an expression of personal excellence of character. In nursing, caring is the central virtue that initiates and molds action. To express the virtue of caring, an ethical standard is required. Since virtues
are dispositions to act in an excellent manner, excellent acts must be
specified (Beauchamp & Childress, 1983). It is the ethic of care that
determines the excellence of action. In contrast to the ethic of care, the
virtue of caring is a standard of excellence in being.

In his theory of virtue, Meilaender (1984) links action with character, doing with being. A reciprocal relationship is identified in which
being shapes doing and doing shapes being. When caring is identified
as the central virtue in nursing, this relationship becomes meaningful
to the educator. In professional behavior, the ethic of care shapes and
influences the professional community's definition of virtuous caring.
Conversely, the virtue of caring shapes and influences how the ethic of
care is expressed on a personal level.

If a goal of nursing education is to develop the personal dimension of
caring, the concepts of care and virtue are useful in the effort. One
method of ethical inquiry enables the nurse educator to link ethics with
virtue. Specifically, the field of virtue ethics is helpful in understanding how and why nurses select between alternative actions when a decision with ethical care content is required.

THE SCHOLARLY STATUS OF VIRTUE ETHICS

For Western culture, the Sophists of ancient Greece were the initial philosophers on the topic of virtue (McGreal, 1970). Plato (a non-Sophist), and his writings on the teachings of Socrates, revised the Sophists' teaching. In his *Republic* (1888), Plato claimed that virtue is the wisdom of one who discovers the forms and ideas of the good and is drawn to them so that conscious action in opposition to the ideas is not possible. Plato identified three natural virtues: wisdom, freedom, and temperance. In Plato's *Protagoras,* through the use of Socratic irony he hints that virtue can be taught.

Aristotle added the idea of two kinds of virtue: intellectual and moral. Intellectual virtue can be taught, but moral virtue is learned by habit (McGreal, 1970). Slaate (1988) credits Aristotle with developing the concept of virtue as an excellent state of character. Excellent states of character make an individual good. Such states also make a person do their work well (McGreal, 1970).

Classical virtue ethics stresses the primacy of the actor in the process of making ethical decisions. The character of the agent as a virtuous person demands right action. Theoretically, unethical behavior results from the actor's lack of excellent character—that is, virtue. Conversely, ethical behavior is the result of the decision-maker's excellence of character (Meilaender, 1984).

Several philosophers, writers, and theologians have been influential in the fall of virtue ethics from mainstream ethical thought. Adam Smith and David Hume and the rise of empiricism were the harbingers of its fall (Blum, 1980). Their ideas, written in the mid-eighteenth century, stressed the centrality of sensate experience. Because much of what virtue ethics had to say about human choice was not perceptible to the senses, it was not considered to be sound epistemologically.

Later in that century, Immanuel Kant advocated the primacy of the nature of the act in determining the morality of action. He is credited with initiating the thinking that led to deontology (Slaate, 1988). The focus of morality shifted from the actor to the act.

The ethics of Eric Fromm and John Dewey identified a third focus of morality, the outcome of the action (Slaate, 1988). Such views are utilitarian or pragmatic. An ethics based on these ideas determines right action in terms of right results. The character of the actor was further devalued.

In the mid-twentieth century, John Fletcher took a most diametrical position. Fletcher (1966) stated that there are no normative standards or virtues. In Fletcher's system, the unique nature of each situation is the focus for determining the morality of the act. Situation ethics completely rejects the idea of a moral excellence appropriate in all situations. This method of inquiry defines the standard of excellence in the changing context. The nature of the actor is subordinated to the characteristics of circumstance.

These and other philosophers created an atmosphere in which the discussion of virtue ethics was virtually eliminated from general discourse on ethics. Walton (1986) states that virtue is alien in the context of contemporary ethics. Duty-based ethical theories prevail in the contemporary system. Universality is desired. By contrast, virtue ethics deemphasizes duty and emphasizes the personalistic aspect of ethics (Walton, 1986).

Virtue ethics, however, is experiencing a renaissance. One reason for its revival is the growth of biomedical ethics. Fry (1988b) states that vulnerable individuals should expect moral excellence in the actions of health care professionals. Media attention to the unethical practices of key professionals in contemporary society has also brought moral excellence into vogue. Meilaender, Brody, and, to some extent, Fry see the field as an exciting area for discourse on ethics.

Beauchamp (1982) argues that the chasm between action-based and character-based ethical inquiry is not as wide as believed. Brody (1988) advocates that the most enlightening method of inquiry includes aspects of virtue ethics as well as deontology and utilitarianism.

Even though virtue ethics can make important contributions to the understanding of ethical care decision making, many questions regarding this method of inquiry remain. The relevance of the concept of virtue in the nursing education setting also raises questions.

Two major questions come to mind. One is rhetorical. Can virtue be taught? The other is more practical. If so, what are the appropriate instructional methods? The following section focuses on a possible answer to the second question.

VIRTUE, CARING, AND TRADITIONAL INSTRUCTION IN NURSING

The answer may be found by examining contemporary ethical instruction in nursing. The predominant texts in nursing ethics reveal the problem.

The field of nursing ethics, like so many other areas of inquiry in nursing, has been permeated with thinking from a biophysical or medical model. Fortunately for the discipline and the profession, nursing is making progress in developing and reconceptualizing its body of knowledge. Nursing has recognized that knowledge of nursing phenomena derived from and conceptualized within a medical, biophysical model is seriously flawed. Why then do leading nurse ethicists conceptualize nursing ethics as a subfield of biomedical ethics?

Most textbooks identify special areas of ethical dilemmas in nursing. Interestingly, the common dilemmas mentioned are genetics and biological revolution, contraception, sterilization, abortion, euthanasia, chemical control of human behavior, consent and refusal of treatment, and issues of death and dying. With the exception of the latter, such lists point to the role of the medical model in current thinking in nursing ethics.

Such dilemmas are examples of biomedical ethics, not nursing ethics. Nurses encounter such dilemmas while practicing in settings in which decision power rests with a physician. In such situations the nurse has little freedom for making choices. If freedom of choice is not present, wherein lies the ethical content?

To conceptualize the phenomena of nursing ethics within such situations and using principles operative in them as the essential dynamics of ethical decision making in nursing is flawed. It is the same type of faulty reasoning that nurses sought to correct when the use of medical diagnoses was replaced with nursing diagnoses. One answer to the question would be to reconceptualize nursing ethics as the ethics of care. Development of the personal dimension of caring is more realistically achieved in this new view of nursing ethics.

Another obstacle to instruction in virtue consists of the methodology commonly used in nursing ethics courses. The typical instructional technique presents the student with some ethical principles and then exposes them to a series of dilemmas. The focus is on dissecting ethical decisions and justifying them using moral arguments. Meilaender points out the incompatibility of such a method with instruction in virtue (1984).

According to Meilaender (1984), these methods teach the student to analyze arguments, not to evaluate moral stances. He claims that experiences in using theoretical propositions cannot teach virtue. Only instruction in a set of moral habits or ways of being can achieve the goal of instilling virtue. Technical expertise in analysis does not impart virtue. Lilla (1981) describes the method of ethical dilemma/decision analysis as a "rather peculiar sort of philosophical discourse which allows the student to make sophisticated excuses for their actions" (p. 4).

Stocker (1973) provides a strategy that is more compatible with the teaching of virtue. He recommends agent evaluation as a valid exercise in the classroom discussion of ethical decision making. Both act evaluation and agent evaluation are necessary to complete instruction in ethics.

Meilaender (1984) attacks another commonly used strategy in moral education. Value clarification is not effective as a method to teach virtue. Value clarification assumes moral neutrality and virtue ethics requires a moral stance. When value clarification is used as the major instructional strategy, character development proceeds no farther than clarity regarding existing inclinations. Value clarification assumes that cognitive clarity and consistency result in exemplary behavior. Meilaender stresses the weakness of such an assumption. He claims that instruction in virtue requires a transformation of a way of being. Whether or not transformation is the best choice of words on Meilaender's part, it is clear that value clarification is inconsistent with basic assumptions in virtue ethics. It is not what is required to teach the virtue of caring.

Teaching the virtue of caring as a central element in professional decision making requires new instructional strategies. These strategies must be compatible with the philosophical base of virtue. Incorporation of virtue ethics as an instructional method through use of agent evaluation is one such strategy. Others need to be developed and refined. The following discussion presents some nascent directions for developing these strategies.

TEACHING STRATEGIES TO DEVELOP THE PERSONAL DIMENSION OF CARING

Plato (1888) developed a scheme for moral education. The first stage consisted of telling stories that bring to mind thoughts and examples of moral virtue. This was to develop a love for what is good. The second stage involved study in disciplines where personal opinions do not matter. Appropriate disciplines are those in which a fact is a fact, for example, mathematics. This was to discourage vanity. The final stage was the introduction of the dialectic.

One creative way to incorporate Plato's thoughts for moral education into nursing education involves three strategies. Nursing programs could structure repeated contacts between the nursing faculty and the student very early in the educational process. During the freshman and sophomore years these early meetings could present thought on and examples of the virtue of caring and the ethic of care. The faculty would relate personal experiences in which they practiced according to the ethic of care. The desired result is an aspiration to be caring on the part of the student.

Another implication is that concrete information on health care provision should precede any material on ethical decision making. This would roughly correspond to the second phase of Plato's process.

Last, the use of dialectic as a method of inquiry could be used in the final courses in the curriculum. However, to be consistent with the concept of virtue, use of the dialectic would entail identification by the student of opposite positions in an ethical care dilemma. The student would have to take a stance and support it while realizing the effect that the opposite stance is having on his or her thinking.

Meilaender (1984) views the structuring of collegiate education as crucial to the teaching of virtue. Accordingly, the university should be a place where the pressure of solutions is subjugated to the experience of the mystery of being. In such an environment the teaching of virtue is an extended conversation between the student and teacher in which conscience is instructed. He bemoans the trend for universities to produce products. Watson (1988) also laments the same trend in nursing education. She challenges educators to emphasize "the subjective, contextual, dialogic, and values-driven" nature of nursing (p. 423). Nursing curricula must be anchored in the liberal arts. Such emphasis promotes the development of the virtue of caring.

The most difficult problem in teaching the virtue of caring effectively originates in the theorized relationship between doing and being (Meilaender, 1984). Practicing according to the ethic of care requires the virtue of caring. But one can only become virtuously caring by practicing according to the ethic of care. This circular pattern is confusing. Meilaender (1984) suggests a solution.

In his book on the theory of virtue, Meilaender advocates that the student be required to act according to an ethical standard of behavior. (In nursing the standard would be the ethic of care.) By conforming or shaping action to a standard of excellence the student begins to shape character into excellence as well. Stein (1986) agrees that the focus should be on behavior. Habituation leads to the development of a caring person. This is consistent with Aristotle, Meilaender, and McGreal. Fowler (1986) claims that virtue is learned by habituating and practicing right action. Meilaender goes as far as to say that even forced adherence to right action develops virtue. He does admit, however, that progress under such conditions is slow. In the brief time that the student nurse spends in coursework at a university it is unlikely that forced adherence will have much success in developing virtue. However, habituation, practice, and clear expectations for excellence are useful ideas.

Developing the personal dimension of caring in the nursing student requires many opportunities to practice the virtue of caring. Clinical experiences need to be selected and structured to facilitate the expression of excellence in caring by the student. If the theorized relationship is true—that is, that being shapes doing and doing shapes being—the student needs a substantial number of clinical experiences. The ethic of care should be the standard for evaluation of student clinical performance.

CONCLUSION

Care is the essence of nursing. The centrality of the concept demands that it permeate all aspects of inquiry and education in nursing. Much debate has focused on the doing of care. It is now time to investigate the being of care. In this effort no philosophy or theory should be dismissed without thorough examination.

One way in which the being of care can be identified and developed is by conceptualizing caring as the dominant virtue within professional nursing. This conceptualization requires that the personal dimension of care be explored.

The field of virtue ethics has much to contribute to the understanding of the personal dimension of action. Within the framework of virtue ethics as applied to nursing, care is an ethic, a standard to which nursing actions are compared for excellence. Caring is viewed as a personal and professional virtue. When a nurse possesses the virtue of caring, aspiration to act in a manner consistent with the ethic of care is ensured. Virtue claims that to be is to do. A virtuously caring nurse will demonstrate care. The concept of virtue provides a way to integrate the total person into the professional role.

The question "Can virtue be taught?" is pertinent. Most virtue ethicists agree that it can and give important ideas on how virtue may be taught. The most common recommendation is that the method and the framework used to teach virtue be consistent with the basic assumptions of a theory of virtue.

Within nursing education, content in nursing ethics must be oriented to the ethics of care. Furthermore, the educational programs should be structured to provide early faculty-student interaction, followed by general education courses, culminating in exercises in the dialectic.

Clinical experiences should be plentiful and focus on practicing the virtue of caring. In the classroom less emphasis should be placed on dissection and more on analysis of ethical dilemmas and decisions. Virtue ethics should be included as a method of inquiry. The emphasis should be shifted to the evaluation of moral stances.

Both the concept of virtue and the use of virtue ethics as a method of inquiry have limitations. Both focus on the personal aspect of the agent. The broader familial, social, and cultural aspects of care are not well served by them. To guarantee that an ethic of care is linked with virtue in a broad sense, personal virtue needs to be conceptualized as having a basis in the cultural belief systems and world view of the actor.

There is also an inherent danger in using some of the strategies compatible with instruction in virtue. The educator must not confuse accountability or adherence to a standard of excellence with conformity in approach or expression. If such confusion occurs creativity in practice will be suppressed. Perhaps the most appropriate method in nursing is to promote creativity in expression of virtue while facilitating adherence to the ethic of care. Use of the concept of virtue in nursing education would be an ill-fated event if it returned us to the task-focused, rigid, perfectionistic methods of nursing's distant past.

Much discourse remains before a definitive statement regarding the validity of conceptualizing the personal dimension of care within the framework of virtue and virtue ethics can be made. There are many areas for further study. An exhaustive debate on whether virtue can be taught is necessary. Further identification and definition of instructional strategies is required. More important, a full explication of the nature and meanings of care must be achieved. When the standard of excellence (care) is clear, students are provided with a more tangible way of being to which they can aspire. Without this full clarity, talk of virtue is meaningless.

Such questions demonstrate the stimulating nature of the fields of virtue and virtue ethics. Nurse educators should investigate the relevancy of these ideas. Formulation of a theory of virtue within nursing just might point the way to development of a professional who unequivocally demonstrates excellence in practice.

REFERENCES

Banner, W. A. (1968). *Ethics: An introduction to moral philosophy*. New York: Scribner.

Beauchamp, T. L. (1982). *Philosophical ethics.* New York: McGraw-Hill.

Beauchamp, T. L., & Childress, J. F. (1983). *Principles of biomedical ethics.* New York: Oxford University Press.

Blum, L. A. (1980). *Friendship, altruism and morality.* London: Routledge & Kegan Paul.

Brody, J. K. (1988). Virtue ethics, caring and nursing. *Scholarly Inquiry for Nursing Practice: An International Journal, 2*(2), 87–96.

Dent, N. J. H. (1984). *The moral psychology of the virtues.* New York: Cambridge University Press.

Fletcher, J. (1966). *Situational ethics.* Philadelphia: Westminster Press.

Fowler, M. D. (1986). Ethics without virtue. *Heart and Lung, 15*(5), 528–529.

Fry, S. T. (1988a). The ethic of caring: Can it survive in nursing? *Nursing Outlook, 36*(1), 48.

Fry, S. T. (1988b). Response to virtue ethics, caring and nursing. *Scholarly Inquiry for Nursing Practice: An International Journal, 2*(2), 97–101.

Gaut, D. (1988). A philosophic orientation to caring research. In M. M. Leininger (Ed.), *Care: The essence of nursing and health* (pp. 17–26). Detroit: Wayne State University Press.

Leininger, M. M. (1988). *Care: The essence of nursing and health.* Detroit: Wayne State University Press.

Lilla, M. (1981). Ethos, ethics and public service. *The Public Interest, 63*(1), 4.

McGreal, I. P. (1970). *Problems of ethics.* Scranton, PA: Chandler.

Meilaender, G. C. (1984). *The theory and practice of virtue.* Notre Dame, IN: University of Notre Dame Press.

Plato (1888). *The republic.* Oxford: Clarendon Press.

Simon, Y. R. (1986). *The definition of moral virtue.* New York: Fordham University Press.

Slaate, H. A. (1988). *A critical survey of ethics.* Lanham, MD: University Press of America.

Stein, A. P. (1986). Teaching nurses to care. *Nurse Educator, 11*(6), 4.

Stocker, M. (1973). Act and agent evaluations. *Review of Metaphysics, 27*(1), 42–61.

Walton, D. N. (1986). *Courage: A philosophical investigation.* Berkeley: University of California Press.

Watson, J. (1988). Human caring as moral context for nursing education. *Nursing and Health Care, 9*(8), 423–425.

16

Theoretical Directives for Care Value Conflict Resolution

Nancy A. O'Connor

One critical challenge in nurse practitioner (NP) education today is to discover ways of maintaining and further developing the students' identity as nurses within this new context of practice. Throughout the 25 years of the NP movement, variability in medical versus nursing role orientations has been common. So prevalent is this issue that Thibodeau and Hawkins (1988) have developed an instrument to quantify the degree of NP orientation toward a nursing or medical model of practice. Loretta Ford (1985), an early pioneer of the NP movement, finds the failure of NPs to remain nursing identified "worrisome" (p. 17) and enjoins NPs to "resolve their identity crisis by joining the family of nursing" (p. 18).

The situation in NP education is analogous to the situation in generic nursing education; in both, the emphasis on care knowledge and caring practices has lagged behind more medically and technologically oriented knowledge. Leininger (1986) has identified several "care resistance factors" (p. 6) that explain this failure to recognize care as the "central and distinct phenomenon of nursing" (p. 1).

This line of reasoning thus posits that a critical indicator of the achievement of and development thereafter of a nursing identity, whether in generic or graduate nursing students, is proficiency in care

189

knowledge and caring practices. Indeed, a 1986 government report on the quality of care delivered by NPs documents that differences in consumer satisfaction with NP- versus MD-delivered primary care lie in the "personal interest exhibited, reduction in the professional mystique of health care delivery, and amount of information conveyed" by the NP (Jacox, 1987, p. 263). These characteristics of NP care can be readily recognized in the care constructs of interest, involvement, sharing and health consultation, health instruction, and health maintenance acts explicated by Leininger (1981).

My experiences in nursing education and service as a nurse practitioner underscore the importance of care value conflict identification and resolution in the formation, maintenance, and growth of nursing identity within students. Those who identify and work through these conflicts within the supportive and facilitative context of nursing education forge a stronger nursing identity evidenced by an increasing caring expertise. How then can nurse educators cultivate and nurture the students' developing nursing identity? Direction has been sought from two theoretical models.

Care value conflicts arise from the diversity of care values within students, between students and care recipients, between personal and professional, between institutional and professional, and between institutional and societal care values. This diversity of care values magnifies the care value conflict potential of the nursing student and can thus serve as an impetus for choice and affirmation of salient caring values, an important step in nursing identity formation. Conversely, failure to identify the care value conflicts and to work toward their viable rapprochement could relate to less favorable consequences of conflict experience such as apathy, withdrawal, or hostility (Deutch, 1971) that could be directed toward care values. Leininger (1974) conducted an exhaustive interdisciplinary review of the conflict literature as relevant to the health professions. Her definitions of conflict and conflict resolution have been adopted here. She defines conflict as "opposing viewpoints, forces, issues, and problems which confront individuals, groups and institutions having been generated from a variety of international and external personal and group forces" (p. 8). She further defines conflict resolution as the "variety of methods and strategies used to resolve opposing individual, group, and social system forces with varying degrees of beneficial and less beneficial outcomes" (p. 9). The potential for diversity to underlie care value conflict potential between professionals and recipients of care within diverse cultures is central to Leininger's (1988) sunrise model of cultural care diversity and universality. In fact, a prediction would follow from the theory that cultural care diversity is related to care value conflict. Cultural care diversity is described as "the variability of meanings, patterns, values, or symbols of care that are culturally derived by humans for their well-being or to improve a human condition or lifeway or face death" (1988, p. 156).

Furthermore, Leininger's cross-cultural care research has thus far demonstrated more care value diversity than universality across cultures. Ray's research on institutional caring (1984) has also demonstrated care value diversity within a hospital or institutional culture and has highlighted the conflict potential for nursing within hospital culture: "By attempting to seek more advancement, recognition, and economic gain within or outside the hospital, conflicts and contradictions have emerged among the caring ideologies of nurses, the institution, and the dominant cultural system" (p. 109). By means of conflict resolution, Ray does not lament the fact that bureaucracy is impeding the attainment of nursing's altruistic care values; instead she calls for a "synthetic" blend of bureaucratic caring with nursing's "ethico-spiritual-humanistic caring" (p. 110).

Another theoretical context for exploring the concepts of diversity, conflict, and conflict resolution is McDonald's (1986) philosophical inquiry into the normative basis of culture. He develops the concept of culture as normative, as contrasted with both subjective and empirical accounts of culture and cultural phenomena. His normative account of culture finds that the meaning of a cultural phenomenon is displayed in the norms, rules, and values that govern but do not dictate people's ways of thinking and acting. This account grounds meaning *in* these norms, rules, and values and *not* in an external natural process (as would an empirical account) or in an internal mental process (as would a subjective account).

McDonald's argument is formulated with reference and direct analogy to the later work of Wittgenstein, who posited the idea of *language* as normative. Based on the normative concept, McDonald develops an analogy between learning a foreign language and learning about cultures other than our own. He points out that we first learn meanings of foreign words by bringing them into relation with words in our own language. More broadly, he develops the argument that what is meaningful to us will always be what is familiar to us. Therefore, we ought first to cultivate a consciousness of our own perspective and a knowledge that this perspective is based on the norms and values of our own culture. Cultivating this consciousness frees us from investing our own cultural presuppositions with an absolute status.

Although not completely commeasurable, the work of Leininger and McDonald share certain similarities in their direction for care value conflict resolution. First, similarities are noted in their views of culture. McDonald's (1986) normative concept has just been described. Leininger describes culture as "the learned, shared, and transmitted values, beliefs, norms, and life practices that guide thinking, decisions, and actions in patterned ways" (1988, p. 156). Therefore, both hold a view of culture as neither subjective nor empirical but normative. Second, both scholars advocate the cultivation of an awareness of one's own cultural perspective, along with the development of an understanding that one's perspective is culturally given. However, neither adopts a stance of cultural determinism but instead speak of norms in the sense of a "moving reference point" (McDonald, 1986, p. 1) and as dynamic structures. Nonetheless, it is clear that for both, cultural beliefs, values, norms, and practices (Leininger, 1988) or actions (McDonald, 1986) are not structures that can be cast off at will. Rather, they are integral to the person. Striving for a critical consciousness of one's own culture *as cultural* is seen by McDonald to "free us from imbuing our own perspective with absolute status" (1986, p. 7). This same critical cultural consciousness is seen by Leininger (1988) to enable culturally congruent nursing care. Can it also enhance the meaningful teaching and learning of care phenomena? Let us now further explore directions for nursing education provided by Leininger's theory.

Leininger's (1981) distinction between generic and professional nursing care and her three nursing care decisions and actions; namely, cultural care preservation/maintenance, accommodation/negotiation, and repatterning/restructuring are germane. *Generic care values* can be seen as the familiar care values of which a critical cultural consciousness should be cultivated in generic nursing students using a process of cultural care preservation and maintenance. In the education of the nurse practitioner, *generic professional nursing care values* can serve as the familiar ground. At each level of education, a new dimension of professional nursing care values can be projected against the familiar ground of the preserved and maintained personal and professional cultural care values. Proceeding from this familiar cultural consciousness, the nursing student is free to negotiate or accommodate diverse care value meanings in a process of conflict resolution. The cycle would close with the students' repatterning or restructuring their care values to reflect a preserved heritage, a contextually sensitive presence, and an on going commitment to the culture of nursing within which the new care value structure was formed.

One final, serious implication for care value conflict resolution can be drawn here from Leininger's (1981) work. Because it is possible and highly instructive to view care value conflict resolution as an intrapersonal and interpersonal process, we must remember that the origins of the conflicts are not limited to these spheres. Recall that conflicting care values are also found at the institutional, professional, and societal levels. Therefore, their resolution should also be pursued at these levels and is clearly the responsibility of the discipline of nursing.

REFERENCES

Deutch, M. (1971). *The resolution of conflict.* New Haven, CT: Yale University Press.

Ford, L. C., & Silver, H. H. (1985). Perspectives 20 years later from the pioneers of the NP movement. *Nurse Practitioner, 10,* 15–18.

Jacox, A. (1987). The OTA report: A policy analysis. *Nursing Outlook, 35,* 262–267.

Leininger, M. M. (November 1974). *Conflict and conflict resolutions: Theories and processes relevant to the health professions.* Paper presented at the ANA Advisory Council Meeting, Kansas City, MO.

Leininger, M. M. (1981). *Caring: An essential human need.* Thorofare, NJ: Slack.

Leininger, M. M. (1986). Care facilitation and resistance factors in the culture of nursing. *Topics in Clinical Nursing, 8*(2), 1–12.

Leininger, M. M. (1988). Leininger's theory of nursing: Cultural care diversity and universality. *Nursing Science Quarterly, 1*(4), 152–160.

McDonald, H. (1986). *The normative basis of culture.* Baton Rouge: Louisiana State University Press.

Ray, M. (1984). The development of a classification system of institutional caring. In M. M. Leininger (Ed.), *Care: The essence of nursing and health* (pp. 95–111). Thorofare, NJ: Slack.

Thibodeau, J. A., & Hawkins, J. W. (1988). Developing an original tool for research. *Nurse Practitioner, 13*(7), 56–59.

17

Using the Arts in Clinical Practice

Silvia Prodan Lange

> The spectacle has begun
> Stay or run
> If you run, you may be sighted and
> cited for leaving the scene of a spectacle
> If you stay, look! Look out!

The creative arts used in clinical practice include drawing, painting, photography, dance, music, drama, and poetry. I will use examples from my own nursing experiences with patients on psychiatric units—acute, long term, day treatment, and outpatient. The creative arts have also been used with other patient groups including children, older persons, rehabilitation units, pain management, those with cancer and substance abuse, those who are dying, and those left behind.

An art, photography, brought me to the University of Colorado for my undergraduate work. In looking at college catalogs, I was captivated by photographs of the Rockies and especially those mystical rock formations, the Flatirons, in Boulder. Fortunately, the University of Colorado is also one of the top nursing schools, especially in what is now called the "psychosocial aspects" of nursing. No wonder the Center for Human Caring was started here.

"As the twig is bent, so grows the tree." My undergraduate experience helped to shape me for my professional career. Two teachers were outstanding—Dorothy Gregg and Catherine Norris. Years later, when we worked together on a project to define mental health content for baccalaureate programs, Kay said that she was the first mental health integrator and I was the first mental health integration student (Carlson & Blackwell, 1978). And I'm still learning!

THEORETICAL FRAMEWORK

The basic concepts I learned in undergraduate and graduate school were modified or reinforced by mentors, colleagues, students, and thousands of patients. These simple but significant fundamental ideas are adapted from Ruesch (1961):

- The nurse/patient relationship develops through interaction and is accessible to observation, examination, and modification.
- Communication is the process by which one person influences another through a continual exchange of expression, reception, and evaluation of behavior. Therapeutic communication differs from ordinary communication in that there is an *intention* to bring about a change in the system and manner of communication.
- Nonverbal communication includes aspects other than words such as body action, gestures, speech patterns, dress, posture, inanimate objects, and use of time and space.
- The arts are powerful and meaningful expressions of human experiences, conflicts, and dreams. Although primarily nonverbal, they can be talked about, which increases their therapeutic potential.

Throughout time human beings have expressed themselves through art, music, dance, drama, and poetry. Following World War Two, the creative arts were developed into therapies that were added to treatment programs for psychiatric patients and other groups. Each specialty has been professionalized with required educational sequences, certification, and national conferences and journals. Nurses can use these modalities without being artists or activity therapists themselves.

In general, the creative arts as therapies are used to foster self-awareness and personal growth. They help to identify and resolve emotional conflicts. They may help to clarify diagnosis and communication styles. For example, the subject that a person draws is important, but also meaningful is how—position on the paper, color, size, emotional accompaniment, how the person reacts to compliments or comments. Kivick and Erikson (1983) identified seven properties of artistic activity as related to psychiatric patients.

Activity vs. Inactivity

It is through activity that individuals create, express, and recreate their relationship to our multifaceted world. The extremes are found: withdrawn, immobile, mute persons to those frenzied with agitation and restlessness. Drawing, painting, and sculpture can be done with others or by oneself. Music can soothe or stimulate, calm or excite. Disturbances of activity are particularly addressed through dance and drama.

Lawfulness vs. Unpredictability

Part of reality testing is to have a reliable perception of both personal strengths and weaknesses along with a grasp of environmental conditions such as rules and consequences. Through working with art materials or the discipline of a musical instrument, persons learn what works and what doesn't. They learn how to be effective, how to persevere, how to fail and to succeed. Even the time set aside for a group activity can be part of a structure that can be counted on.

Imagination vs. Overconcreteness

The creative arts provide multiple opportunities to leap yet be grounded. They allow so-called grownups to be children again and to play in a safe, joyful way. They help us to re-create ourselves.

Sensory Expressiveness vs. Strictly Verbal Expression

The arts are powerful and persistent expressions of the human experience. Long before verbal and written words, humans drew animals on their cave walls, chanted and danced to prepare for battle or celebrate the seasons. The shaman played a healing role through drama and action. Although all people can benefit from sensory experiences, two groups of patients seem particularly helped—those who are withdrawn, mute, nonverbal, or highly symbolistic and those who are overly verbal with high levels of intellectualization.

Concentration vs. Distraction

Involvement depends on the ability to concentrate, to pay attention. Many psychiatric patients have major problems with preoccupation or short attention spans. The creative arts help to focus and to screen out competing stimuli.

Catharsis vs. Inhibition

The creative arts help persons to experience and express internal perceptions and feelings rather than repressing, denying, distorting, or inhibiting them. Many patients show disturbed and destructive behavior—the acting-out of emotions. Or they can be so out of touch with feelings that they seem mechanical, the "computer personality." The arts evoke powerful emotions and though providing channels of expression keep them from being overwhelming. They help to alleviate guilt and to express anger in appropriate ways.

Mastery vs. Helplessness

This polarity is one most persons experience periodically along the life span. Patients are usually very high on feelings of helplessness and very low on mastery. Yet, to be able to leave a treatment setting and stay out, one must develop some degree of personal control. The creative arts foster mastery by encouragement to follow through on such things as finishing a painting or sculpture, practicing being assertive through role-playing, and completing a group project. For long-term institutionalized patients, the idea of "learned helplessness" is all too applicable. Persons who learn how to express themselves through the arts have found creative outlets and socially valuable skills.

CLINICAL EXAMPLES

I have used the creative arts in my nursing practice in a variety of ways. Most of these examples come from groups. The advantages of working with patients in groups are the power of group dynamics and the opportunity to experience similarities and uniqueness. The arts serve as equalizers with persons who may have divergent backgrounds. In addition, groups are both time- and cost-effective.

Visual Arts

Early in my nursing career, I spearheaded a small redecoration project on the ward and wrote it up as "The Therapeutic Collage" (Prodan, 1959)—a metaphor for the blending of the talents of the patients in an art project using magazine covers. Over the years I have collected a variety of pictures, drawings, and photographs that I have used in many ways. They serve as informal projective tests or triggers. I've used them to help people identify assets and goals—"Pick a picture that represents something about yourself that you like; pick one that shows something you'd like to change." At Christmas we've had symbolic gift giving where patterns of giving and receiving emerge. The beginning to a standard relaxation exercise is, "See yourself in a calm, safe place in nature." If a person has difficulty with visualizing, these pictures can help. Years later the therapeutic collage emerged in a different form—stitchery. I started a huge wall hanging of free-form flowers and leaves that new patients added to. When we hung it in the lobby, we titled it, "I Never Promised You a Rose Garden." I've used my collection of cartoons about a wide variety of human foibles with patients and students. I also developed a series of word doodles, diagnostic conundrums that require an oblique, right-brain approach to solve them (Lange, 1981) (see Figure 1).

Photography—another visual art—can be helpful; for example, pictures of a patient's early family and important relationships. I've used videotapes of informal groups as well as specific groups such as assertiveness training and psychodramas. A spin-off of my interests led to my workshop on poetry films at the first International Imagery Conference in New Zealand—a program titled "The Cycle of Death and Birth."

Dance

My first contact with psychiatric patients was before my psychiatric nursing rotation; I was a volunteer at weekly square dance sessions. One partner was from the "violent" ward. He walked off the floor and left me when the call was "bump-si-daisy" (bump hips). At the time, I wondered whether our caller should modify his calls in light of possible conflicts or whether it was better for the patients to deal with what most of us do, the "bump-si-daisys" of life.

In graduate school, I wrote my thesis on nonverbal communication. To sensitize myself, I enrolled in a physical education course in modern dance. The teacher was an European traditionalist who couldn't believe it when I told her why I was taking the course. "You want to dance with the

Figure 1

These perplexing puzzles are word doodles—visual puns. Figure out the Sx, Hx, Rx, Px, etc.

Hint: P(1)ay attention to the graphics, location, size, word in a word. This feature was first published in the *Journal of the Operating Room Research Institute.*

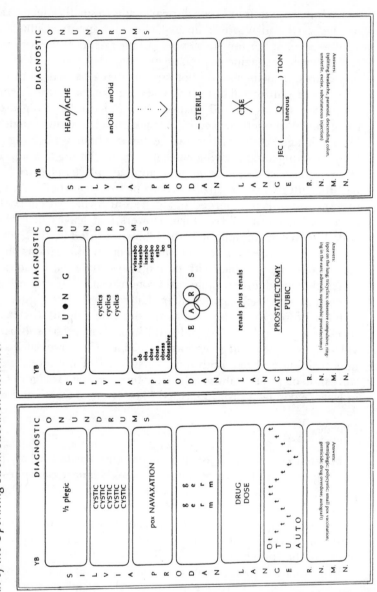

insane?" And I did. I went to work at Boston State Hospital where there were 3,000 patients in 1960. The director of nursing, Lillian Goodman, was a creative administrator. She allowed me to choose my assignment. I picked a back ward where there had never been a professional nurse. The patients were profoundly regressed and socially isolated; they and the staff were institutionalized, a phenomenon known as mutual withdrawal.

One of my stipulations for working on the unit was that I would have nursing students assigned there. So when I started a ward dance group, they took an active part. That's another benefit for using the creative arts in a group setting—there are multiple opportunities for teaching students and staff. The purpose of the group was to encourage social interaction through dance and music. We moved individually, then in pairs, and finished up in a circle. I varied the rhythms and numbers with a balance of repetition and novelty. Two months before Christmas our dance group was asked to take part in the hospital-wide holiday program. Despite our stagefright, we did a great job. And every year at Christmas when I hear "Jingle Bell Rock," I think back to when, yes, I *did* dance with the insane.

Drama

Psychodrama is a treatment approach in its own right that provides a meaningful arena to deal with past, present, and future experiences. It does require specialized training. Nurses can become effective members of a psychodrama team (Lange, 1968). I've played many different roles including being a patient's ulcer. Role-playing and role reversal are psychodramatic techniques which can be very helpful in other situations. Guided imagery and visualization contain aspects of drama. I've used these with individuals and groups for stress management, weight control, and pain management. For one young woman with severe agoraphobia I tape-recorded our walks from her apartment, down the elevator, and to my office so that in time she could come by herself with the help of her Walkman and her personal guided fantasy. I've used my psychodramatic background to volunteer at a mock trial of malpractice involving suicide. I scripted and videotaped typical group situations to test a support group training project.

Poetry

Poetry is a bridge between nonverbal and verbal expression. Like many other health professionals, I've written poetry for my personal pleasure and as a creative outlet. When I was teaching at Seattle University, I asked students in psychiatric nursing to write haiku as a means to communicate about themselves and their patients in a succinct, creative way (Lange, 1964). I've led poetry groups where we have read classic poems about a theme such as loneliness. In other groups we wrote poems; once I played a tape of wolves howling and the poems ranged from fear to friendliness. Occasionally, we put out a newspaper where the poems were published as a group effort. On several occasions I have written poems for persons that I was seeing in individual psychotherapy and then given the poems to them. I was an invited participant at a national poetry conference talking about poetry as a healing art.

CONCLUSION

Nurses and nurse educators who use the arts in their clinical practice can expect to learn about and deal with issues of particular concern both to themselves and the profession. These include creativity, competition, ambiguity, body image, and self-disclosure. They can expect to be surprised. The use of the creative arts can produce powerful and meaningful results with profound levels of communication. These can be healing for the individual and the group.

Now, for my finale, I will make a spectacle of my self. A spectacle is an attention-getting, eye-catching dramatic public display. Originally, this piece chronicled the evolution of women psychotherapists. Later, I realized it had relevance for millions of women around the world. And for this conference, it is applicable for health professionals, and especially nurses.

Act I

This is my dancin' outfit (Isn't it cute?)
These are my dancin' shoes (Don't you just love 'em?)
I would do anything you asked me
I would do *anything*, and I mean anything *you'd* choose
Including abuse
Which led to the blues

Act II

This is my running outfit
These aren't my running shoes (I can barely stand up in them, much
less run or dance in them)

Can I do anything I want to?
Can I do anything I choose?
Including to lose?
Which leads to the truth!

Act III

This is my sexy outfit
These are my sexy shoes
I can do anything *I* want to
I can do anything (well, almost) I choose
Including refuse
Which leads to confuse

Act IV

Now here's the hard part; here's the scary part
'Cause this is my naked outfit
And these are my naked shoes
I know that *you and I* can do anything we want to
I know that *we* can choose
And I know that it's better in twos
Which leads to . . .
The End . . . or . . . Is it the Beginning?

REFERENCES

Carlson, C., & Blackwell, B. (Eds.). (1978). *Behavioral concepts and nursing inter-vention* (2d ed.). Philadelphia: Lippincott.

Kivick, H., & Erickson, J. (1983). The arts as healing. *American Journal of Orthopsychiatry, 53*(4), 602–618.

Lange, S. P. (1964). Haiku in psychiatric nursing education. *Nursing Outlook, 12,* 52–53.

Lange, S. P. (1968). Nurse participation in action techniques. In *American Nurses' Association Clinical Sessions 1968*. New York: Appleton-Century-Crofts.

Lange, S. P. (1981–1983). Diagnostic conundrums. *Journal of the Operating Room Research Institute*. Monthly feature.

Prodan, S. (1959). The therapeutic collage. *American Journal of Nursing, 59,* 1288–1289.

Ruesch, J. (1961). *Therapeutic communication*. New York: Norton.

BIBLIOGRAPHY

Arieti, S. (1976). *Creativity: The magic synthesis*. New York: Basic Books.

Bailey, L. M. (1985). Music's soothing charms. *American Journal of Nursing, 11,* 1280.

Berne, E. (1953). Concerning the nature of communication. *Psychiatric Quarterly, 27,* 185–198.

Blatner, H. A. (1973). *Acting-in.* New York: Springer-Verlag.

Clarke, L. M. (1982). Art therapy: A learning experience for students in nursing. *Journal of Nursing Education, 21*(6), 4.

Cook, J. D. (1981). The therapeutic use of music: A literature review. *Nursing Forum, 20*(3), 252–266.

Johnson, D. R. (1985). Expressive group psychotherapy with the elderly: A drama therapy approach. *International Journal of Group Psychotherapy, 35*(1), 109–127.

Johnson, J. L., & Berendis, C. A. (1986). Arts and flowers: Drawing out the patients' best. *American Journal of Nursing, 86*(2), 164–166.

Karasu, T. (Chair). (1984). The creative therapies. Psychodrama. In *The psychiatric therapies.* Washington, DC: American Psychiatric Press.

Koch, K. (1977). *I never told anybody: Teaching poetry writing in a nursing home.* New York: Random House.

Lange, S. P. (1970). Esalen . . . and afterward. *Nursing Outlook, 18*(6), 33–35.

Lange, S. P. (1978). Shame, hope, transactional analysis, and nursing. In C. Carlson & B. Blackwell (Eds.), *Behavioral concepts and nursing intervention.* Philadelphia: Lippincott.

Lerner, A. (Ed.) (1977). *Poetry in the therapeutic experience.* New York: Pergamon Press.

Ludwig, A. (1989). Reflections on creativity and madness. *American Journal of Psychotherapy, 43*(1), 4–14.

Malamud, D. I., & Machover, S. (1965). *Toward self-understanding: Group techniques in self-confrontation.* Springfield: Thomas.

Oiler, C. (1983). Nursing reality as reflected in nurses' poetry. *Perspectives in Psychiatric Care, 21*(3), 81–89.

Prodan, S. (1959). *An exploratory study of the use of nonverbal communication in identifying a theme in a nurse-patient relationship.* Unpublished master's thesis, University of Washington, Seattle.

Rosen, E. (1957). *Dance in psychotherapy.* New York: Teachers College Bureau of Publications.

Ruesch, J. (1952). The therapeutic process from the point of view of communication theory. *American Journal of Orthopsychiatry, 22,* 690–670.

Ruesch, J. (1955). Nonverbal language and therapy. *Psychiatry, 18,* 323–330.

Ruesch, J. (1957). *Disturbed communication.* New York: Norton.

Schloss, G. (1976). *Psychopoetry.* New York: Grosset & Dunlap.

Schutz, W. (1967). *Joy: Expanding human awareness.* New York: Grove Press.

18

Deciding to Care: A Way to Knowledge

Patricia Moccia

Nancy Reagan and I are different. First, the obvious: she appears anorexic and I obviously do not and she's a little shorter. Then there are the less obvious differences of preference: she likes red and I prefer blues and purples. Other differences you can't see but can surmise by our choices: she likes the West Coast and I prefer New York, she takes rich macho business men as her heroes, and I prefer women and men who work incessantly to express their passions thoughtfully and respectfully, whether the passions be for art or human service or building a closer world community.

The list of differences could go on, but I think they can be summed up in one slogan, she would have you "Say no to drugs" and I would have you say "yes." That generic decision, whether to say yes or to say no, presents itself in every interaction of our lives, no matter how significant or how mundane the decision. Yes or no. Yes, we are connected to what is presenting itself as our reality, or no, we are not connected. Yes, the reality is our reality, or no, it is not.

Saying "yes," attending to what is in front of us, such is our decision to care. Saying "no," not attending, separating ourselves, is deciding not to care.

Saying yes connects us to our reality in new ways. Saying yes, then, will lead to more knowledge about our worlds. Saying no cuts us from knowing the connections that tie us together. Saying no limits our knowledge of our relationships; distorts and deforms our reality.

Back to Nancy Reagan and me, for more clarification before one of you runs off to find the Denver police, or runs up here to offer me some drugs to test my rhetoric. There is a second difference in the yes or no answer to drugs. Nancy is focused on the individual, on the individual interaction, the individual decision, the individual responsibility, the individual dissociating herself from what is being offered. My yes is not to the buying or selling of drugs, but to the context, to the complex of relationships that manifest itself in the offer to sell drugs and the complex of relationships that lead to the yes or no decision to buy them. I urge you to attend to such relationships, for example, to the relationship of class between the seller and the potential buyer, the relationship of gender and race, of power and domination.

If you were to say yes rather than no to the situation as distinct from the individual interaction around drugs, you might learn several things. For instance, first, you might learn about yourself, what you value, what you fear. You might learn the glorious feelings of autonomy and self-determination as you say yes to the context but decline the drugs. You might learn of your complexity, your many thoughts and feelings that pervade the interaction. Then, you might learn of the peasants of South and Central America who work as laborers in fields where drugs are grown and harvested—the question of the value of human life. You might also learn of the relationships of power and exploitation between governments.

Decide to care by saying yes to attend to the context rather than the individual and you will know more than before the interaction. As you are well aware, saying yes rather than no to context and relationships preeminently, rather than to individualistic cause and blame, is not the approach that we have been taught and not the mode into which we have been socialized. But, I suggest to you, such is the approach that is needed if we are to create the knowledge we so desperately need in order to be a healthy community.

CONNECTED

I'd like to share some thoughts, then, about the realities that present themselves to us, the moments of experience that call for our decisions.

Did you know that Einstein once called our sense of being separate an "optical delusion" for he knew that we were all connected in quite profound ways. Our spirits, souls, emotions, and physical being are connected within ourselves in ways we know of, but cannot name. We are born into a social world of ongoing activity that precedes our awareness of being. To be precise, our social being *allows* our individual being. We come to know our own selves and our position within such a world through still more social interactions. Our experience of being, within the time and spaces of the eternal process which we find to be our own, such experiences are *connected* to the others, to their experience of being *connected* also to the unfolding of nature's experience of itself—and all is *connected,* in quite profound ways, to the evolution of being itself.

To understand otherwise is to be misled and fooled, as in a carnival funhouse, as Einstein warns, by an optical delusion. And yet we build our world on such delusions, structure our societies and our communities on such delusions, attempt to live our lives, seek to understand ourselves and our neighbors, try to live and to care for ourselves and for our friends, within such delusions. But the delusions can only delude for so long, the forces of reality eventually break through even the most grand delusion. Eventually the reality of our interrelatedness, of our *connectedness,* becomes clear to even the most delusional among us.

For example, although the ideology of the United States would have us believe that we are an independent and separate state, with our borders protected against all but who and what we allow to enter, the windborn fallout from the nuclear accident at Chernobyl in the Soviet Union forces us to acknowledge the power of nature to unite nations.

We might delude ourselves into a middle-class complacency that drugs and violence are parts of others' lives but are not *connected* to our own. Until, that is, the reality of our connectedness breaks through, as the paper reported last week, when the stray bullets of drug dealers shattered the windshield of a congressman riding with his family on the streets of Washington on his way to a White House reception. Or as it does when we ask our 8-year-olds the age-old question "What did you learn in school today" and they reply that "Johnny or Janie got in trouble for bringing a bag of crack capsules and a gun to class."

We might delude ourselves into thinking that we are not *connected* to teenage pregnancy, that it has nothing directly to do with us, as we plan our careers and listen to the biological clock, and structure our lives and our work so successfully that we have it all, and we take pictures of the family at Christmas that look like Ralph Lauren ads. Until—another story from the papers—we are hurrying late one evening to our car in the parking lot and a young girl steps from the shadows, thrusts a baby in a dirty blanket into our arms, and says "Please take her, I can't take care of her."

At that moment across the lines that divide us, across the barriers of class and race that separate our societies, the reality of our connectedness literally forces itself onto and into our lives. No matter if we take the baby home, to a shelter or social service agency, or brush past them and into our car, the *reality of our connectedness* was there to see and feel and not to be denied.

We might even comfort ourselves with liberal delusions that it is enough to be so saddened and sympathetic about the poverty rates and the illiteracy rates in this country that we donate money to a host of organizations and lobby for governmental programs. But because the lives of the poor and uneducated seem so far removed from our own, so unconnected, we assure and delude ourselves and our friends that such actions are all we can do or all we ought to do. After all, we argue to ourselves in our own defense, we have to live our own lives and dedicating one's self to the social good is an adolescent idealism that is most appropriate for the first job after college but certainly not the third or fourth position into one's career.

The forces of reality break through these delusions of separateness when the fact that 32.5 million people live in poverty in this country, that millions of these are children, that 2 million of those who live in poverty hold full-time jobs, comes dramatically home to us in the current situations in our health care system. Without access to preventive and primary care services, the poor come to our hospitals in distress with multiple systems compromised; once there, they further exhaust already exhausted resources. In legitimate need of relief from the suffering, illness, and disease that accompany the fact of being poor in America, these individuals are filling hospital beds in our communities.

We might be able to delude ourselves into acting as if the lives and illnesses of the poor are separate from our own, that we are not connected, until we wake up in the middle of the night in our own acute pain, and we spend hours waiting to be cared for in an overcrowded emergency room. Or spend days on a stretcher in the halls outside an emergency room because there are no beds available upstairs for they are filled with the poor, with victims of violence, with people with AIDS, with substance abusers. The dismal joke in New York and other cities is that you can tell the person with real political influence, not by who can get tickets to a Knicks game, or a seat at the opera, or a pass to the Van Gogh exhibit at the museum, but by who can get a bed in any hospital, not even the best hospital, but any hospital when they need it.

We might trick and delude ourselves into believing that we can be isolated from the troubles around us, that we can provide for our families all they might need, until you and I cannot have a nurse come to our homes to care for our parents and we cannot find a long-term care facility for the friends we know who are living and dying with AIDS. Why? Because the money in health care has been tied to hospitals, connected to the hospital through a weave of an almost insatiable greed for profit, a medical arrogance and domination, an institutionalized set of patriarchical relationships of domination and submission, a weave that reproduces and extends itself.

At these moments of our own need, our own pain and fear, our own frustration and despair, at moments such as these our connections become painfully clear, our delusions break down. This optical delusion that is our bubble of self-deception violently bursts into a quiet vapor of realization. In the moment of such realization, as we face the reality of our connectedness, the experiences of being separate are exposed as foolish fancy at best and dissociative states at worst; as disturbances in our relations with our worlds that threaten all our relations; as mental aberrations destructive for our health and our lives and destructive for the whole of humanity.

Given that these optical delusions of separateness have become so much a part of our lives that we mistake them for reality, is it any wonder that the carnival's funhouse has become our house of terror. As in the funhouse, or as in our dreams, yet we struggle to find our way home, or out of the delusion, or pull ourselves back from sleep, to rescue ourselves from the hell that T.S. Eliot describes, where nothing is connected to nothing.

How is it that we have come to accept such delusions as real? Surely we are not dupes, yet we have been misled; we have become so separated from our realities that we live ignorant of our profound connections. And, in turn, we are profoundly impoverished by our ignorance. Even the most wise among us too often cannot see reality for delusions.

In a poem titled "Power," Adrienne Rich (1974) talks about Madame Curie:

> Today I was reading about Marie Curie
> she must have known she suffered from radiation sickness
> her body bombarded for years by the element
> she had purified
> It seems she denied to the end

the source of the cataracts on her eyes
the cracked and suppurating skin   of her finger-ends
till she could no longer hold   a test tube or a pencil
She died a famous woman   denying
her wounds
denying
her wounds came from the same source as her power.

And so I ask you to follow this poet's direction, I ask you to look to the source of our wounds for the source to our healing. Look to these optical delusions for insight about the nature of our reality. Look to these moments of feeling separated, of being divided, of experiencing our distance one from the other; look to these wounds for the power we need to know another reality, the real connections.

I ask you to consider that deciding to care, by saying yes rather than no, is a way to counter these delusions. Deciding to care by saying yes rather than no and attending to context rather than individuals is a way to bring reality to the surface, a way to reinforce reality's natural tendency to intrude into our delusions.

Deciding to care is an approach that would have us search for the connections in our separations. Deciding to care will help us to create the knowledge that will make explicit the hidden and profound connections of our lives, and in the making of such knowledge, the decision to care will strengthen our connections.

But you will obviously ask me how are we to do this, how are we to care in a society that neither teaches, nor allows, the space for caring. And by the way, you might also say, you have convinced us of the need to care, but before we jump right into it, what exactly do you mean by caring, define your terms, sister.

Caring is such a popular concept these days. The term itself is so much a part of the vernacular that I'm certain that those who have devoted significant portions of their life projects to thinking about caring, caring about caring, writing about caring—these adventurers in caring get a little nervous, I'm certain. About how it's being bandied about; how, perhaps, it's being misunderstood, misused, and in places even abused.

In what has become an immediate classic, *The Primacy of Caring*, Patricia Benner and Judith Wrubel (1989) use the word "caring" to mean being connected, to have things matter. Benner and Wrubel argue that caring fuses thought, feeling, and action; it fuses knowing and being and so is primary to our existence. Caring sets up what matters, it creates possibility, it creates connection and concern, it creates the actual sharing of help, allowing one to give and allowing another to receive.

Bernice Fisher and Joan Tronto (in press) viewed caring as "a species activity that includes everything we do to maintain, to continue and to repair our world so that we can live in it as well as possible." Fisher and Tronto identify specific preconditions that influence the degree, quality, and extent of caring—time, material resources, knowledge, and skill.

Although differing in degree and emphasis, and in Fisher and Tronto differing in class analysis, each of these women who have shared their ideas and feelings with us through their writings and through their lives, each of their expositions underscore that caring *assumes* and *allows connection*. Such an understanding of caring enhances our chances of building on the experience of such connections rather than on the optical delusions of separateness. By presupposing connection rather than isolation as a defining characteristic of the species, each offers a way out of the house of terror; each offers an alternative to Eliot's wasteland where nothing is related to nothing; each points the way to our knowledge and to our power.

Now that we have some definitions, how and where are we to begin, you say to me again. Jean Watson presents us with "Human Caring: A Public Agenda," Wingspread paper (1989). Drawing on the work of Chinn, Gadow, Quinn, Benner, and Ray, Watson is clear in her call for caring as a public agenda. Watson is clear in sharing what is needed to pass a certain threshold of consciousness, to push away the rock of conformity. Watson generously shares her clear direction of how to get where we want to be from this point at which we find ourselves, how to counter our delusions: "Caring like freedom and love is created everyday in ways small and demanding, tedious, painful, and endured like time itself."

Commit yourself to counter delusions. I ask you to consider how to care, how to learn to say yes, how to learn to see contexts and relationships rather than immediate and individual situations. Perhaps you might consider developing for yourself what Janice Raymond describes in her book *A Passion for Friends* as a "creative habit." Quoting Mary Daly, Raymond reminds us that to develop such "creative habit" calls for arduous practice and thoroughly repeated acts.

For whatever reasons, we have chosen education as our life's work. Here, we have incredible opportunity to counter delusions in our interactions with our students, to establish the climate within which both teacher and students can practice such creative habits. Within our experiences with students we can say yes to the context of the situations; we can explore the power relations between us; we can explore the relationships of class and race that separate us and connect us; we can explore the process of the experience; we can say yes, and claim the experience as our own.

In our daily experiences with students, whatever the context, whatever the course, whatever the clinical setting, we can develop creative habits, practice them over and over until our first approach to any situation is to say yes rather than no. Practice them over and over until every individual situation is attended to in the context of its relationships. Practice them over and over until our delusions of being separate no longer sustain our structures and our organizations; repeating yes and focusing on relationships until such an action becomes our creative habit; saying yes to the student-teacher relationship itself, by focusing on how we are connected rather than on how we are different.

And so deciding to care is not only a way to knowledge, it is a way out of the wasteland, a way out of the house of terror, a way out of our delusions. It is a way to community and, so, to health and wholeness. Develop the creative habit of looking to how we are connected to the drug pusher rather than to how we are separate; develop the creative habit of looking to our relationship to the poor rather than how we differ; develop the creative habit of claiming our reality of and accepting our relationship to what presents itself as reality; develop the creative habit of saying yes rather than no; develop the creative habit of deciding to care in each and every of your interactions throughout the day.

Be careful with yourself while striving to say yes and attend to context at every moment throughout the day. At every decision point there will of course be times when you say no and when you cannot see the context for the immediate. To those moments, I ask you also to say yes, claim them as your reality, attend to their connections with the times you've said yes, care for yourself by deciding to say yes to yourself, care for yourself by attending to the context of your decisions.

I read a line somewhere that's either attributed to Fidel Castro or was said about him: "Every person is an answer to a question. Victory to those who say YES."

REFERENCES

Benner, P., & Wrubel, J. (1989). *The primacy of caring: Stress and coping in health and illness.* Menlo Park, CA: Addison-Wesley.

Fisher, B., & Tronto, J. (in press). Toward a feminist theory of caring. In E. Abel & M. Nelson (Eds.), *Circles of caring.* New York: State University of New York Press.

Raymond, J. G. (1986). *A passion for friends.* Boston: Beacon Press.

Rich, A. (1984). Power. In *The facts of a doorframe.* New York: Norton, p. 225.

Watson, J. (1989). *Human caring: A public agenda.* A paper presented at the Wingspread Conference: Knowledge About Care and Caring, Racine, WI.

19

A Caring Community

Sonya Hardin

The purpose of this chapter is to increase knowledge of community health nursing from a human science perspective. Polkinghorne (1983) defines human science as an inclusive approach to human phenomena that uses multiple systems of inquiry. Hence, nursing as a human science uses multiple modes of knowing and views caring as the essence of nursing. Specifically, the mode of inquiry that I will discuss is aesthetics. Aesthetics opens nursing up to the possibilities and the imagination that will be needed to creatively increase nursing's knowledge in the next decade.

Martha Rogers' (1970, 1980) conceptual system provides a world view from which development of a caring community is explicated. A piece of visual art, "A Caring Community," provides the focus of an aesthetic representation of caring. An aesthetic description of the visual art reflects congruency with Rogers' system.

Rogers' system can facilitate caring as an expressive form of nursing. Although the proposed model of a caring community may not be useful to practice directly, it provides a substantive base for research and theory development that can enlighten the knowledge base for practice (Quillin & Runk, 1983). The potential also exists for construction of discernible hypotheses that require innovative methods of validation within a community study. These innovative methods could provide a different way of understanding community.

217

COMMUNITY

Rogers' world view proposes a better understanding of community. In this, *community* is a large human energy field that has a unique pattern. As a number of human energy fields evolve, each with its own unique pattern, they merge into a larger energy field. Community presents itself as this *large* human energy field.

The concept of community includes three aspects:

1. The exchange of energy patterns among two or more human energy fields within an integral contextual setting.
2. Within a contextual setting, the exchange of energy patterns that are spatial (territorial) and conceptual (rules, sanctions) fields of interactional activity delineating open boundaries.
3. The exchange of energy patterns between two or more human energy fields that evolve into an understanding of the common need for the whole.

The exchange of energy patterns provides a unique meaning of community for each human energy field.

Community is understood as a unified whole possessing integrity and manifesting characteristics that are more than and different from the sum of parts. Community as a human energy field is open and it is engaged in a continuous interaction of exchanging matter and energy with the environmental field. This continuous interchange of matter and energy between the community and environment is the basis of each human energy field's unique perception of community. This mutual changing is innovative and it marks the life process of the community unfolding. Although the life process of the community evolves through time and in a space-time continuum, it can also be understood as a symphony of rhythmical vibrations oscillating at various frequencies.

In fact, community projects into the past and future. It is a four-dimensional human energy field of a world of neither space nor time. Community, itself a four-dimensional field, is embedded in a four-dimensional environmental field. As such, community is the relative present for the whole.

Community exists in a probabilistic universe and is subject to Rogers' three principles of homeodynamics. The principle of *helicy* allows community to be understood as a rhythmical ordering of life. The principle of *resonancy* makes explicit that community is a wave pattern that continuously changes from lower to higher frequency wave patterns according to the ordered arrangement of the rhythm of the community energy field and environmental field. The principle of *integrity* is the evolving life process of the community and environment.

The primary postulate of the conceptual development of a caring community is that a harmonious life process rhythm relates to the concept of caring. Caring is a pattern manifested in the human energy field of the community nurse: caring is the essence of nursing. This pattern of caring can be understood as an action (Gaut, 1986) which is present if, and only if (1) the human energy field has identified a need for care and has knowledge of what to do for another human energy field; (2) a human energy field implements an action intended to serve as a means for positive change; and (3) the welfare of the other energy field is used to justify the choice activities identified as caring. For caring to occur, an attitude of respect for the other must be present. Caring is an example of a symphonic exchange of energy in a harmonious arrangement like that reflected in Rogers' principle of synchrony. In this case, change in the human field depends only on the simultaneous state of the environmental field at any given point in space-time (Rogers, 1970, p. 98). Caring as a symphonic exchange of energy is a matching in a segment of time. It is a synchronic interaction described by Wertz (1979, p. 89) as verbal and nonverbal components interwoven in an interactive dance of great elegance and rhythm.

Caring, as defined by Gaut (1986), reflects an action that requires a human energy field to be sensitive to the needs of others (the environmental field). It requires being at the right time and right place for the welfare of others. This synchrony emerges as nurses act and administer to the community.

The community is the heart or, rather, the focus of a community nurse. The nurse is an environmental energy field in the community. As an environmental energy field the nurse provides care (a pattern of the human energy field) to the community. Caring occurs when the nurse and community evolve as a whole; maintenance and promotion of health evolves from the caring action of the nurse. The nurse seeks to promote symphonic interaction between community and environment, strengthen the coherence and integrity of the community energy field, and direct and redirect patterning of the community and environmental fields to maximize health potential (Rogers, 1970). The community and nurse are in a continuous progress of evolution toward both diversity and complexity of the pattern.

Community must be attended to by the nurse as a dynamic evolutionary process. Since the total pattern of events at any given point in space-time provides the data of nursing diagnosis (Rogers, 1970, p. 125), nurses have the capacity to establish harmony in the community and to provide care.

AESTHETIC DESCRIPTION

An aesthetic description of a caring community is congruent with Rogers' conceptual system. Using metaphor in conjunction with Figure 1, A Caring Community, one can understand something "complex, contextual, and unknown about caring in an almost unconscious flash of light" (Watson, 1987, p. 11). The metaphors were chosen through a creative process of attempting to find new methods to express the covert, intangible, tacit, expressive dimensions of caring in community nursing (p. 11). However, this creative process requires an imaginative thought process of the reader and viewer of this text and the visual piece of art in Figure 1; the materials of the work of art do not, in themselves, embody its meaning. The work's significance depends, rather on the manner in which the materials are organized (Phenix, 1964, p. 156). Visual arts are "arts of space." A full visual understanding is not achieved instantaneously. Rather, the model is revealed step by step in time, as one visually explores the work (p. 153).

Figure 1* is a two-dimensional representation of a three-dimensional piece of visual art which portrays an expressive form of caring in a community. Beginning inside the model and dancing back and forth from inside to outside, the heart signifies the community. The heart symbolizes the center of human activity, the life process.

The life process of many human energy fields evolving together as community is central to the focus of nursing. The heart is covered with white gauze. The white gauze symbolizes the texture and pattern of waves characteristic of the community energy field: if two waves reach a certain spot exactly in harmony with each other, their vibrations reinforce each other; they produce a greater pattern than either would alone. This greater pattern is a white light. But, if the two waves arrive completely out of step, their vibrations oppose each other; the net result is zero disturbance, darkness or blackness (Hoffman, 1959, p. 37).

---

*Please note that the representation of the figure as printed in this book may not exactly mirror its description.

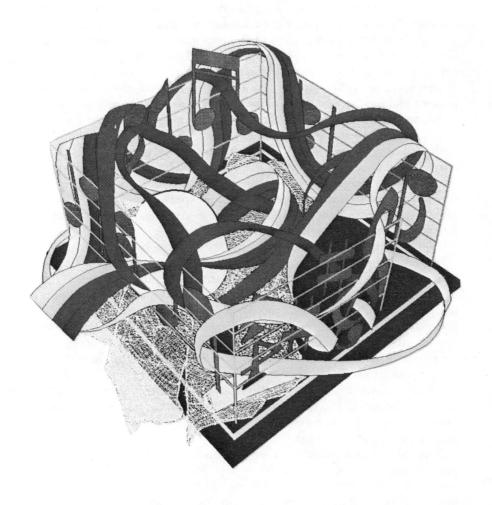

Hence the black background of this art work symbolizes waves (energy fields) opposing each other. The white gauze stretching out over the white heart into infinity represents waves (energy fields) in harmony with each other. If a community exists as a white light then harmony is present for a context of caring.

The environmental field is represented as a scale of music. It is through the interexchange of the community energy field and environmental field that manifestation of nonrepeating rhythmicities evolve. Community is in open interaction with the environmental field; through this open interaction harmony exists as caring. The community and environment are wave patterns denoted by the musical notes. This wave pattern changes continuously from lower frequency, longer wave patterns, to higher frequency, shorter wave patterns. This rhythm is a mutual process of change. The musical score expresses harmony of the caring community as a matrix flowing over time. Harmony is the balance between opposing forces of the universe. The meaning of music is most intimately connected with the rhythmic sense, which in turn is directly related to the fundamental human experience of time. Time is measured by movement and rooted in the human heart as the regular pulses with recurrent cycles (Phenix, 1964, p. 147).

In the original three-dimensional piece of art, the broken mirror was scattered on the black background. The broken pattern of mirror cannot be seen in the two-dimensional representation of Figure 1. However, the broken pattern of mirror serves two purposes: the mirror represents the process of reflection and the concept of four-dimensionality. The process of reflection allows each experience of community to be unique for the individual. Through reflective experience, the community is able to transcend; transcendence enables the community to know. Because of the community's ability to transcend, the whole can make decisions about truth and falsity, beauty and ugliness, right and wrong, holiness and profanity (Phenix, 1964). The community is able to know the past, present, and future in a relative moment. Hence, at any moment, the past, present, and future exist.

The mirror is a reminder that community is four-dimensional. A present point in time is relative to each human energy field in the community; the mirror can create a sense of movement, of resonance, of process. A sense of movement directs the imagination toward the possibilities of the future. Anticipation of the future is a way of acknowledging the concept of time; the reflection from the mirror provides an ascent into transcendence (Turner & Bruner, 1986).

The harmony of community exists because of nurses' capacities to care. This is seen in Figure 1 as the ribbons emerging from the community and environmental field as shades of grey. The ribbons emerge as an universal whole and then separate. This separation represents many modes of caring. The colors in the original piece were chosen to express forms of caring that occur in different intensity. When light waves are of low frequency, they correspond to red light. As the rate of vibration increases, the color changes to orange, then to yellow, and so on right through the colors of the rainbow (Hoffman, 1959, p. 13).

Caring is a dynamic pattern emerging out of the community and environmental energy field. It is a manifestation or behavior of the nurse that permeates the whole. The harmonic rhythm of the whole emerges out of the dynamic pattern of caring. Hence, caring contributes to the balance and harmony of the community.

Aspects of this model have been described, but the whole, not the aspects, is the focus of our understanding. The whole is a view of the harmonious interconnection between the human energy field (community) and the environmental field. Each human energy field of the community energy field transcends to the whole as a source of uniqueness for each individual. Hence, each individual has a unique understanding of a caring community.

In sum, the model is an aesthetic presentation of nursing in the community. The work of art as a whole is the bearer of artistic import, as is a painting or a drama (Langer, 1979, p. 201). One may isolate certain beauties of the work, but its meaning reflecting Rogers' conceptual system is not determined and supported without the context of the written description. The work will hold a different meaning without the text. One might consider this a limitation of the model. Yet the visual form is capable of allowing the profession of nursing the opportunity to appreciate caring and to see it in a new way with or without text. This model highlights the need to use intuition, creativity and aesthetic perception in nursing educational activities.

Gendron (1988) states that the aesthetic way of knowing is relatively undeveloped in nursing education; Travelbee (1971) suggests the use of parables; Gendron (1988) suggests the use of visual diagrams, visualizations, collages, and imaginative stories to apprehend aesthetic forms of caring. The model used in this chapter is an example of the technique of transforming Rogers' world view into a visual art form. Aesthetic forms of knowing enhance the value of aesthetic attitudes and intuition in nurses (Gendron, 1988). Yet other ways of knowing should not be neglected in nursing educational methods. Instead, a blend is needed that will increase holistic understanding and awareness.

REFERENCES

Barrett, E. (1989). A nursing theory of power for nursing practice: Derivation from Rogers' paradigm. In J. P. Riehl-Sisca (Ed.), *Conceptual models for nursing practice* (3d ed.). Norwalk, CT: Appleton & Lange.

Cerilli, K., & Burd, S. (1989). An analysis of Martha Rogers' nursing as a science of unitary human beings. In J. P. Riehl (Ed.), *Conceptual models for nursing practice* (3d ed.). Norwalk, CT: Appleton & Lange.

Chinn, P. L., & Jacobs, M. K. (1983). *Theory and nursing: A systematic approach.* St. Louis: C. V. Mosby.

Chivington, P. (1983). *Seeing through your illusions.* Boulder, CO: G-L Publications.

Dossey, L. (1982). *Space, time and medicine.* Boulder, CO: Shambhala Publications.

Ference, H. M. (1989). Comforting the dying: Nursing practice according to the Rogerian model. In J. P. Riehl, *Conceptual models for nursing practice* (3d ed.). Norwalk, CT: Appleton & Lange.

Gendlin, E. (1981). *Focusing.* Toronto: Bantam Books.

Gendron, D. (1988). The expressive form of caring. *Perspectives in Caring Monographs.* Toronto: University of Toronto.

Hoffman, B. (1959). *The strange story of the quantum.* New York: Dover.

Langer, S. (1979). *Philosophy in a new key: A study in the symbols of reason, rite, and art.* Cambridge, MA: Harvard University Press.

Malinski, V. (1986). *Explorations on Martha Rogers' science of unitary human beings.* Norwalk, CT: Appleton-Century-Crofts.

Meleis, A. I. (1985). *Theoretical nursing: Development and progress.* New York: Lippincott.

Phenix, P. (1964). *Realms of meaning.* New York: McGraw-Hill.

Pibram, K. (1971). *Languages of the brain.* Englewood Cliffs, NJ: Prentice-Hall.

Polkinghorne, D. (1983). *Methodology for the human sciences: Systems of inquiry.* New York: State University of New York Press.

Quillin, S., & Runk, J. (1983). Martha Rogers' model. In J. Fitzpatrick & A. Whall (Eds.), *Conceptual models of nursing: Analysis and application.* Bowie, MD: Robert J. Brady.

Rader, M. (1979). *A modern book of aesthetics.* New York: Holt, Rinehart & Winston.

Rogers, M. E. (1970). *An introduction to the theoretical basis of nursing.* Philadelphia: Davis.

Rogers, M. E. (1980). Nursing: A science of unitary man. In J. P. Riehl & C. Roy (Eds.), *Conceptual models for nursing practice* (2d ed.). New York: Appleton-Century-Crofts.

Rogers, M. E. (1983). Science of unitary human beings: A paradigm for nursing. In I. W. Clements & F. B. Roberts (Eds.), *Family health: A theoretical approach to nursing care.* New York: Wiley.

Rogers, M. E. (1985). In A. I. Meleis (Ed.), *Theoretical nursing: Development and progress.* Philadelphia: Lippincott.

Rogers, M. E. (1986). Science of unitary human beings. In V. Malinski (Ed.), *Explorations on Martha Rogers' science of unitary human beings.* Norwalk, CT: Appleton-Century-Crofts.

Rogers, M. E. (1989). Nursing: A science of unitary human beings. In J. P. Riehl (Ed.), *Conceptual models for nursing practice* (3d ed.). Norwalk, CT: Appleton & Lange.

Sarter, B. (1988). *The stream of becoming: A study of Martha Rogers's theory.* New York: National League for Nursing.

Speilberg, N., & Anderson, B. D. (1987). *Seven ideas that shook the universe.* New York: Wiley.

Talbot, M. (1986). *Beyond the quantum.* New York: Bantam Books.

Travelbee, J. (1971). *Interpersonal aspects of nursing* (2d ed.). Philadelphia: Davis.

Turner, V. W., & Bruner, E. M. (1986). *The anthropology of experience.* Chicago: University of Illinois Press.

Watson, J. (1987). Nursing on the caring edge: Metaphorical vignettes. *Advances of Nursing Science, 10*(1), 10–18.

Weitz, S. (1979). *Nonverbal communication: Reading with commentary* (2d ed.). New York: Oxford University Press.

Whelton, B. J. (1979). An operationalization of Martha Rogers' theory throughout the nursing process. *International Journal of Nursing Studies, 16,* 7–20.

Wolf, F. A. (1984). *Star wave: Mind, consciousness and quantum physics.* New York: Macmillan.

20

Using Photography with Families of Chronically Ill Children

Mary Hagedorn

> Chronic illness is like a piece of sand
> inside an oyster,
> It irritates and creates a pearl,
> Or it just dies.

Kate Wilkinson

This metaphor, expressed by a parent dealing with a child who has a chronic illness, conveys the presence, changes, and outcomes that often accompany chronic illness. "Chronic illness is at the same time a personal misfortune and a sign of progress. No longer illnesses to die of, but still not thoroughly curable, these illnesses become illnesses to live with" (Register, 1987, p. 9).

Gendron (1988) stated that an aesthetic attitude is important when becoming aware of self and others. In perceiving someone or something aesthetically one is able to appreciate a unique or individual quality thereby seeing the person or thing in a new way. Because an aesthetic attitude is important in becoming aware of the self and others, there is an aesthetic character to the practice of nursing. A valuing of an aesthetic attitude and intuition when grasping the gestalt of a patient encounter suggests that more use and development be made of methods in education programs that foster these attributes.

This chapter will introduce a process utilizing photography when interviewing families with chronically ill children. Photography offers an aesthetic approach for nurses that provides new insights and knowledge about subject matter. Collier and Collier (1986) stated that "photographs can be communication bridges between strangers that become pathways into unfamiliar, unforeseen environments and subjects" (p. 99). Thus, photographs can function as starting and reference points for discussing the unfamiliar or the unknown.

Although the camera has been used for collecting visual data for decades in anthropology and sociology, little has been done to explicate the value of the camera in nursing research. The camera as a tool can be equated with the tape recorder commonly used for recording verbatim detail in qualitative research. Photography is an abstracting process of observation but very different from field notes where information is preserved in literal form. Photography gathers selective information, information that is specific with qualifying and contextual relationships that are usually missing from codified written notes (Collier & Collier, 1986). "Photographs are precise records of material reality" (p. 10).

Photography also has a potentially important role in nursing because of its specificity and ability to present interrelated wholes. "Photography can aid in preserving these vivid first impressions in a responsible and usable form" (Collier & Collier, 1986, p. 16). Photographs can also be tools with which to obtain knowledge beyond that provided through direct analysis. They can accurately record materials and circumstances about which we have limited knowledge. Through the practice of photography and the analysis of photographs, another dimension of knowledge and observation evolves that results in the sharpening of our visual senses. The overall objective is to communicate and educate about a phenomenon. Again, photography can aid in preserving first impressions in a responsible and usable form. However, "Photography is only a means to an ends, a holistic and accurate observation, for only human response can open the camera's eye to it's meaningful use in research" (p. 5).

According to Collier and Collier (1986), a series of photographs can make the strongest visual statement about an experience and can be used during a photographic interview process to illuminate the experience. The images captured in photography invite people to take the lead in inquiry, facilitating their discussion of the experience. As such, photographic interviews are not only an experiment in gathering information but also an effort to enrich and extend existing interviewing methodologies.

When using photographs during interviews, the potential range of data enlarges far beyond the photographs themselves. For example, photographs invite open expression, while maintaining concrete and explicit reference points. They can sharpen the memory and give the interview an immediate character of realistic construction. Photographic interviews also offer a unique return of insights that might otherwise be impossible to obtain with other tests or techniques. As a result, the use of a photographic interview can provide a unique methodological approach for investigating an experience (Higgins & Highley, 1986).

In addition, photographs can divert the informant from wandering out of the research area. Photographic interviewing allows for structured conversation without inhibiting the informant (Collier & Collier, 1986). Photographs allow the person to tell his or her own stories spontaneously. Photographs offer fluency and imagery to the interview, an opportunity that can reveal a great deal about an experience. As Goldschmidt and Edgerton (1961) have stated, "Photographs present all elements simultaneously, without differential emphasis, while a statement is by the nature of language linear. The symbolic meanings of the artifacts are themselves significant and . . . their significance is once removed when substituted for by verbal expression" (p. 41). All the rewards of interviewing with photographs stem from the phenomenon and the return of the informant to that familiar image of reality (Collier & Collier, 1986). Photographic interviewing can break through the barrier to enhance communication.

An important consideration in patient photography is the acquisition of proper written consent. A potential risk of patient/family photography results from misinterpretation of the meaning of the photographs.

Photographs can subtly reassert humanistic and compassionate dimensions of health care, dimensions that are seriously endangered by the demands of a highly technological field. Hopefully, through photography, a more sensitized awareness of the human condition can be achieved through viewing and studying visual data. At minimum, the camera can serve as a notebook for recording visual content to facilitate a more thorough analysis by the researcher/observer.

This author utilized photography in a study whose aim was to describe the experience of having a chronically ill child from a parent's perspective. The key elements of photographic interviewing were illustrated in a visual photographic journey with a set of parents who chose to capture the experience of having a chronically ill child through photographs. These parents revealed a great deal of information about the experience of having a chronically ill child. Had a traditional interview format been followed, however, the information that was revealed might not have been shared.

The chronically ill are still a largely unidentified group within our population (Register, 1987). Chronic illness plagues 10 to 15% (7.5 million) of children in the United States. Twenty-two out of every 1,000 children have 1 of the 11 most common childhood chronic illnesses (Hobbs, Perrin, & Ireys, 1985). These children utilize more than 60% of all inpatient resources (Perrin, 1987). Chronic conditions, though rarely cured, are managed through individual and family effort and diligence (Thomas, 1984). Persons enduring chronic illness cannot discard the sick role. Neither acutely ill nor completely well, the child with a chronic illness and the family must make daily changes in their lifestyle. As a result, chronic illness does not strike just the individual, it strikes the whole family (Futcher, 1988). Patterson (1985) stated that "unlike acute illness where a patient is usually hospitalized and under the direct care of a physician and medical professionals, the chronically ill child spends most of his or her time at home, dependent upon parents or other family members for care and treatment" (p. 75).

Chronic illness may present in many forms. It can occur suddenly or through an insidious process, have episodic flare-ups or exacerbations or remain in remission with the absence of symptoms for long periods of time (Lubkin, 1986). Maintenance of a degree of wellness and self-care is at times difficult. The presence of multiple disease entities complicates the outcome for the child, and makes planning for the future uncertain.

The essence of chronic illness is the challenge of this era for health care professionals and institutions. Chronic illness is increasing in proportion to the earth's population yet neither the public nor health care professionals recognize the full implications of the education, care, training, and financial burdens that confront the family and the child with chronic illness.

If researchers are to learn about issues surrounding chronic illness, however, the common but complex problems of chronic illness need to be studied in an experiential manner. Strauss (1984) stated that, "perceptive eloquent autobiographies by the patients" are the key to understanding the life experiences of the chronically ill (child) (p. 10). With the rise in the number of chronically ill children, it becomes imperative that nursing develop a scientific knowledge base about chronic illness that enables nurses to assist parents in dealing with the necessary complex care. To develop such a knowledge base, Watson (1985) stated that the nurse researcher should:

> choose methods that allow for the subjective inner world of personal meaning to be revealed. Nurse researchers can choose to study the inner world of experiences rather than relying on the outer world of observations (p. 345).

Watson (1985) has described nursing as a human science which views human beings as experiencing beings. "Generally nursing phenomena and the human science perspective of nursing are consistent with the approach that is experiential, qualitative, and contextual" (p. 17).

Moccia (1988) stated that the call and response of an authentic dialogue between a nurse and patient has great power—the power to change the lived experience of both the patient and nurse, to change the situation, to change the world. We often seek the person who really listens to what we are saying, who really tries to understand our lived experiences of the world and who asks the same from us. Bohm (1980) and Newman (1986) both concluded that it is the nurse who is responsible for aiding the person in making sense out of the chaos and disruption that illness can cause. "When we can help create meaning, it is easier to remember why we chose nursing and why we continue to choose nursing despite the underpaid and undervalued job it has become in today's marketplace" (Moccia, 1988, p. iv). A human's need for care demands caring actions on the part of the nurse. Caring is a concern for and is the essence of a helping relationship (Gaut, 1983). Gaut explicates caring as an action which requires nursing to be sensitive to the needs of others.

Paterson and Zderad (1988) proposed that nurses consciously and deliberately approach nursing as an existential experience. Nursing is an experience lived between human beings. Existential experience infers human awareness of the self and others. It calls for a recognition of each person existing singularly in his or her situation and struggling and striving with their fellow persons for survival and becoming, for confirmation, and for existence and the understanding of its meaning. Nursing, of course, is embedded within this human context. As a result, contemporary nursing calls for understanding the mental, emotional, and imaginative feelings of clients. To enhance such understanding, the nurse and patient or group of patients participate in an artistic experience together. In fact, humanistic nursing is itself an art—a clinical art—that is creative and existential. As a clinical art, it involves being with and doing with.

As Watson has so aptly stated (1985):

> An ideal of intersubjectivity (that incorporates subjective-self, human presence and touch and new aesthetic caring processes) is based upon a belief that we learn from each other how to be human by identifying ourselves with others or finding their dilemmas in ourselves. What we learn from other's condition is self-knowledge. We learn to recognize ourselves in others (pp. 59–60).

Many of the questions dealing with human experience lend themselves to research methodologies that may use aesthetic tools as a means of enhancing the interviewing process. Photography is one of those tools. This overview of photography and its uses hopefully challenges other researchers to use photography in their research endeavors.

REFERENCES

Bohm, D. (1980). *Wholeness and the implicate order.* London: Ark.

Collier, J., & Collier, M. (1986). *Visual anthropology: Photography as a research method.* Albuquerque, NM: University of New Mexico Press.

Futcher, J. (1988). Chronic illness and family dynamics. *Pediatric Nursing, 12*(3), 191–193.

Gaut, D. (1983). Development of a theoretically adequate description of caring. *Western Journal of Nursing Research, 5*(4), 313–324.

Gendron, D. (1988). The expressive form of caring. *Perspectives in Caring Monographs.* University of Toronto.

Goldschmidt, W., & Edgerton, R. (1961). A picture technique for the study of values. *American Anthropologist, 63*(1), 26–47.

Higgins, S., & Highley, B. (1986). The camera as a study tool: Photo interview of mothers of infants with congestive heart failure. *Children's Health Care, 15*(2), 119–122.

Hobbs, N., Perrin, J., & Ireys, H. (1985). *Chronically ill children and their families.* San Francisco: Jossey-Bass.

Lubkin, I. (1986). *Chronic illness impact and intervention.* Boston: Jones & Bartlett Publishers, Inc.

Moccia, P. (1988). Preface. In J. Paterson & L. Zderad, *Humanistic nursing.* New York: National League for Nursing.

Newman, M. (1986). *Health as expanding consciousness*. St. Louis: C. V. Mosby.

Paterson, J., & Zderad, L. (1988). *Humanistic nursing*. New York: National League for Nursing.

Patterson, J. (1985). Critical factors affecting family compliance with home treatment for children with cystic fibrosis. *Family Relations, 34,* 74–79.

Perrin, J. (1987). Chronically ill children in America: The case for home care. *Journal of Physicians in Home Care, 5,* 54–62.

Register, C. (1987). *Living with chronic illness*. New York: The Free Press.

Strauss, A. (1984). *Chronic illness and the quality of life*. St. Louis: C. V. Mosby.

Thomas, R. (1984). Nursing assessment of childhood chronic conditions. *Issues in Comprehensive Pediatric Nursing, 7,* 165–176.

Watson, J. (1985). *Nursing: Human science and human care. A theory of nursing*. Norwalk, CT: Appleton-Century-Crofts.

21

The Moral Dimension:
Humanism in Education

Cheryl Demerath Learn

This chapter stresses the importance of and suggests methods for developing a philosophy of education. Humanism, as derived from existential-phenomenological philosophy, is considered as a philosophy of education appropriate for a human caring, practice-oriented program of education for professional nurses.

DEVELOPING A PHILOSOPHY OF EDUCATION

As educators in human care nursing, we must think deeply about the work that we do. Developing a philosophical perspective of education, though not easy, is a moral necessity if a nurse educator wishes to be an effective professional educator. A philosophical orientation gives depth and breadth of meaning and direction to personal and professional endeavors (Osmon & Craver, 1986).

How, then, does one develop a philosophical perspective for an educational program? Does one arbitrarily select a certain framework? Developing a philosophy of education does not mean making an uncritical acceptance of this or that principle or system or school such as Neo-Thomism or the Social Progressive perspective. First, it means making a responsible examination of what the differing philosophies of education offer in light of existing, social, educational, and contextual factors. It means delving into the many philosophical writers in the field of education. Since education is such a vital part of life, almost every philosopher since Socrates has had something to say about it.

Second, it is important to clearly think through exactly what one believes about nursing and nursing education. Most nurse educators have already either consciously or unconsciously developed such beliefs but often have not formalized them (Bigge, 1982). Third, one needs to consider several contextual variables such as the notion of education for a practice discipline, caring, the amount of time that one has students, and the underlying philosophy of the parent institution.

After such thought, study, and reflection most educators find that a certain philosophical approach appears most congruent with their personal beliefs. For example, humanism as derived primarily from the existential-phenomenological philosophies of education best articulated my underlying personal beliefs and was compatible with notions of nursing as a human science based on caring.

Notice the use of the word *primarily*. Educational philosophers have suggested that a responsible eclecticism or emergent synthesis of philosophies of education is important (Bigge, 1982; Osmon & Craver, 1986). No single educational philosophy is ever totally suitable at any particular moment. Thus, one may have to strike out in new philosophical directions, return to the ancients for guidance and wisdom, or look to philosophies outside of one's culture such as Eastern traditions. Regardless of whether one chooses a single educational philosophy in its totality or derives one from the contributions of several philosophies, it is possible to develop a personal educational philosophy that can be supported by its internal harmony and educational adequacy (Bigge, 1982).

THE IDEA OF HUMANISM

Humanism is a notion that, like love, resists classification (Wineberg, 1972). Humanism can be anything that human beings can be. There are many versions of humanism drawn from differing philosophical viewpoints. For this chapter, humanism as an idea and philosophical perspective is drawn from the works of several philosophers of education. One major writer about humanistic foundations of education is Martin Buber (1958), who emphasized the I-thou dialogue that requires mutual respect, dignity, and appreciation of the rich uniqueness of every individual. As Weintrout (1963) states, "This dialogue is basic to his religion, his philosophy, and what he has to say about education" (p. 53).

Morris and Pai (1976) wrote extensively about the educational uses of existentialism and humanism. Freire (1974) contrasted education as liberation with education as oppression. Knowles (1973) explicated the principles of adult education. Weller (1976) wrote about and developed several alternative schools. Whitehead (1967) addressed issues related to the role of the university.

HUMANISM AS A PHILOSOPHY OF EDUCATION

John Dewey (1897) posed five succinct questions in his "pedagogic creed". These questions still offer a framework that is broad enough to provide a useful approach in developing a philosophy of education. According to Dewey, a philosophy of education needs to address five main areas or articles. They are:

1. What are one's beliefs about what education is?
2. What are one's beliefs about what the school (university) is?
3. What are one's beliefs about the subject matter of education, which is Dewey's description of the student?
4. What are one's beliefs about the nature of method?
5. What are one's beliefs about human progress?

In addressing the first question from a humanistic framework, education is primarily self-actualization wherein the whole person is encouraged to grow intellectually, emotionally, and socially in such ways as to be able to deal effectively with life now and in the future (Morris & Pai, 1976). Education, seen as a humanizing process, attempts to counteract the dehumanizing effects of a highly and increasingly technological society. "Humanists emphasize the power and dignity of human beings, the worth of personality and the freedom and responsibility of developing human potential so that people can solve their own problems with reason" (1976, p. 139). A humanistic philosophy of education draws heavily from existentialism, one of the most individualistic of philosophies (LaMonica, 1985). Although there are many different approaches to existentialism, this philosophy is concerned with human longing and search for meaning within the self. An existentially based education assumes the responsibility of awakening each individual to the full intensity of his or her selfhood (Morris, 1966).

The University

What does a humanistic philosophy state regarding the definition of a university? Since few existentialists or humanists overtly answer this question, other sources are utilized. Whitehead (1967), who is generally considered a contemporary realist, thought that the justification for the university was that it preserved the connection between knowledge and the zest for life in the imaginative consideration of learning. Past experience and newer ideas must be welded together in such a way as to create meaning for one's life. For the nursing student, the university should be a place where the student will develop an appreciation for the many dimensions of human experience, including the values, practitioner skills, and attitudes that are essential for the caring profession of nursing (Sakalys & Watson, 1986).

The second and equally valuable function of the university is the social responsibility of the university to provide competent professionals to meet the demands of an increasingly complex society. Whitehead (1967) reminded us that since its earliest days, the university has always had a sense of mission in meeting society's needs for physicians, clergy, and law clerks. Whitehead even maintained that "At no time have universities been restricted to pure abstract learning" (1967, p. 137). In summary, the purposes of the university are two-fold. The epistemological purpose is the bringing together of knowledge and new life for the generation of innovative scholarship. The social quest is the emphasis on education in terms of its contributions toward meeting the professional needs of society.

The Learner

In article 3, Dewey developed his ideas of the subject matter or the student. In a humanistic philosophy of education, it is beliefs about the nature of the learner that are of prime importance. The learner is perceived as one who is valued and who is greater than the sum of his or her parts. A human being is not a determined being nor an organism whose behavior is elicited by external conditions (Sarter, 1987). The learning process is the search for personal meaning in existence and leads toward self-actualization.

If the major goal of such education is self-actualization, then it is necessary to believe that all persons are capable of growth and have the desire to grow. The focus here is on the uniqueness of the individual rather than on the commonalities of the group. There are indications that the varieties of students are increasing in complexity. For example, one could consider age or ethnicity. In many universities, the average undergraduate age is well over 25. Students are often older, have a vast array of experiential and educational knowledge, and frequently have many other roles besides that of student (Kaseworm, 1980). Colleges of nursing are no exception. A university education is becoming more and more available to a broader variety of citizens. No longer is it limited to the white, male members of the upper class. These different students are requiring diversity in methods of teaching and approaches.

The Nature of Method

Dewey's fourth major article concerned the nature of method. In a humanistic, caring educational environment, the nature of method should foster a holistic integration of knowledge derived from many disciplines. The classical liberal arts need to incorporate models of professional education (Sakalys & Watson, 1986). The role of the teacher is to assist the learner in working out the significance of what has been learned in relation to its meaning in the learner's life. This role requires a supportive learning environment characterized by trust, spontaneity, and reward. In such an environment participation by learners needs to be active (Morris & Pai, 1976).

The teacher is to assist the student to become a fully functioning person. Specific methods could include problem-posing and -solving as suggested by Freire (1974), discovery learning, self-initiated projects, and learning to deal effectively with problematic situations through practicums as suggested by Schon (1987). The teacher who is striving to teach in a humanistic spirit needs to have several attitudes. Teachers are to be facilitators of student learning, not simply experts. The teacher is to view self as one possible resource among many others that the teacher makes available for the student to choose from. In contrast with traditional settings, where the teacher is the expert who gives information to the student who is a novice, the teacher is a fellow learner. Freire (1974) contrasted the traditional banking method of education where students are the depositories and the teacher the depositor: "Education must begin with the solution of the student-teacher contradiction by reconciling the poles of the contradiction so that both are simultaneously teachers and students" (1974, p. 59). In contrast, in problem-posing education, both teacher and students join together in posing problems and their solutions (1974). The former is oppressive while the latter can be liberating academically and politically.

Social Progress

In article 5, Dewey's focus is on social progress and the school. What does a humanistic philosophy of education say to us today about social progress? Not as much as might other philosophies of education such as Marxism, Pragmatism, and the Social Progressive movement. Existentialism, as the underlying philosophy of humanism, concentrates on the individual rather than social progress or collective welfare issues. Unlike other philosophies, humanism based on existentialism is not primarily a social philosophy but an individual philosophy. "Society is played down and the individual is emphasized" (McDaniels, 1983, p. 65). Yet there are implications for social progress.

If, as Sartre (1974) stated, existence precedes essence and we are free to construct meaning in any way we see fit, then we are totally responsible for what is or will be. Thus, oppression can be eliminated if we ourselves can become perceptive to all possibilities and encourage our students to become attentive to all possibilities. Freire (1974) argued that the roots of oppression lie in the ability of the oppressor to present a mythological, final picture of reality, whereas an awareness of all possibilities would permit a reality susceptible to transformation. This points to the prospect that we can individually refuse to be what an oppressive society wants us to be and choose change.

Contemporary Illustrations

A recent application of the principles of a humanistic philosophy of education can be seen in the contemporary development of adult education theory. Although there are numerous theories in this emerging discipline, one of the most influential ideas of adult education is Knowles's concept of andragogy (1973), which is the art and science of helping adults learn. In contrast, pedagogy is the art and science of helping children learn. Andragogy rests upon four assumptions about the adult learner:

1. As learners mature, their self-concepts move from dependency to autonomy. An adult who chooses a selected educational experience is self-directing and will respond positively to those situations where the adult is free to assist in decision making and where his or her adult input is valued.

2. As an individual matures, a growing reservoir of experience accumulates which then becomes an increasing resource for learning. Based on this assumption, the adult learner prefers teaching-learning strategies that use and value previously acquired experience.

3. The adult's readiness to learn is often oriented to developmental tasks, which generally involve perception of social role.

4. An adult learner's time perspective is often one of immediate application. Implications for curriculum and teaching suggest an approach where creative solutions to problems would be tried soon after the problem has been identified or posed.

Knowles is not the only adult educator who has incorporated a humanistic philosophical approach in his work. Knowles' work has focused on adult learning in the Western democracies. In a different vein is Freire's work with adult learners in the third world. Freire (1974) focused on liberation through teaching reading literacy to adults. It can be concluded that humanism as a philosophy of education has much to offer educators in various settings where more and more students are and will continue to be adults.

HUMANISM AND HUMAN CARE NURSING EDUCATION

A humanistic philosophy of education has much to offer a human caring, practice-oriented educational context. The implications are broad and will affect all beliefs about education, the university, the student, method, and human progress. Our beliefs about what education is will need to expand and grow. Perhaps the greatest change will appear in the areas of the nature of method. Most readers would agree that behaviorism, greatly used in nursing education, is incongruent with the precepts of human caring and a humanistic philosophy of education. In the effort to move away from behavioristic learning theory, a humanistic philosophy offers choices closer to our understanding of nursing as a human science. According to Bevis (1988), behaviorism supports training, not education. Thus, a humanistic approach contributes to the development of broader educational outcomes than the narrow linear scope of behavioral objectives and encourages the learner to gain knowledge and a depth of understanding on a level greater than skill acquisition.

Why is a humanistic philosophy of education important to nursing? "The human science view of man is the most comparable with the nature of nursing and the processes by which learners achieve practice competencies" (Reilly & Oermann, 1985, p. 18). Sakalys and Watson (1986) describe nursing as a rapidly growing human science that focuses on the human care aspects of individuals and groups of clients. If one of the desired outcomes for graduates of nursing education programs is to have practitioners with a human care philosophy and orientation to practice, then this practitioner must be educated in such a fashion that embodies the student as a whole person of immediate worth.

THE MORAL DIMENSION

If a humanistic philosophy of education and nursing education based on human caring are so compatible, why is it necessary to explore the moral dimension of humanism in nursing education? The word dimension has within its family of meanings not only the sense of perspective but also associations with measurement, especially depth and breadth. Moral refers to the good or bad. Thus, we need to carefully consider the strengths and weaknesses and the depth and breadth of the implications of a humanistic philosophy of nursing education.

Evaluation

Special attention must be given to student evaluation in a humanistic setting. Evaluation is usually perceived as a continuous process of collecting information, considering what has occurred, and judging its worth (Reilly & Oermann, 1985). A philosophy of humanism as the underpinning of an educational program of human care nursing changes our perspective of student evaluation. Due to power issues, the idea of traditional student evaluation becomes a dilemma in a humanistic framework. In a dilemma, one is faced with choices that are equally unfavorable or equally favorable. Because of a variety of interacting elements, uncertainty can prevail (Berman, 1988). We can be torn between the idea of our primary educational values of learner self-actualization and individual freedom and our responsibility to public safety. When compared to students and graduates of other university programs, there is a different moral dimension for nursing students and graduates who work directly with human life and death issues. Society expects us as caring and therefore competent nurse educators to allow into practice only those practitioners who have proved themselves to be safe providers of nursing care. In many other disciplines, the risks with human life are not nearly so great and there is a distancing of time and end results.

A situation where a student has grown self-actualized but our caring professional judgment tells us that this individual may not be a safe clinical practitioner is just such a dilemma. Our caring commitment to society mandates us to graduate safe competent practitioners of nursing. Under the old rules, using external criteria of clinical competence and public safety, we can decisively fail a "weak" student. It is considerably more difficult when we must work with such an individual to mutually resolve such a dilemma. It is to be hoped that in an environment where self-knowledge, mutual trust, and human freedom are predominant characteristics that the student will realize that he or she is not ready or has not grown sufficiently for independent practice at this particular time. Thinking through and reconciling these kinds of dilemmas will not be easy.

Questions and Concerns

Other recent questions and concerns pertain to the implementation or actualization of such thinking. Nurse educators need to seriously consider such questions and issues as:

1. Humanism (overtly or covertly) is a prevailing theme in recent publications on nursing and nursing education (National League for Nursing, 1988). Are we moving in a direction where a humanistic approach is seen as a panacea? We are barely off the good ship behaviorism!

2. Many phrases such as humanistic, existentially based, and freedom are used loosely and generally as though there were one commonly understood meaning to these words. There isn't.

3. Freedom presents some interesting dilemmas. We need to clarify in a humanistic, caring-based nursing educational environment what is meant by freedom and what its implications are. What is freedom? What is license? Is warmth, empathy, personal concern, and freedom sufficient or adequate if we lack direction, normative values, content, or context (Weller, 1978)?

4. Recent articles in the literature have discussed curriculum revolution and revision. If the transformation of nursing education into a human caring context is going to occur, it must be at a depth far more radical than that of the curriculum itself! It may even mean the total restructuring of colleges, schools or departments of nursing as well as the transformation of nursing itself (National League for Nursing, 1988).

5. Given that we can choose change and freedom from oppressive environments, how do we implement these transformations when many of our settings, institutions, and even accrediting regulations contradict the very changes we wish to make?

6. How do we work with students who have already been socialized or oppressed into existing systems of banking education? It is a challenge to undo 15 or more years of such training.

There are no easy answers to these or other difficult questions. It is, however, vital that they be raised to expand the dialogue and clarify exactly what we are about. The answers undoubtedly lie in many places. Some answers may be in new philosophical directions themselves. Some answers will emerge as we implement new human caring educational worlds. Some may come from the ancients as we return to their work for guidance and wisdom to interpret and solve our current and future problems. Some dilemmas that surface may never be resolved (Berman, 1988).

Because we are in a critical era of transition, a study of philosophies of education is an important part of today's educational imperative. In times of great change, it is easy for people to embrace more and more change with little thought to eventual consequences or to resist change and keep old values, no matter what the cost (Osmon & Craver, 1986).

REFERENCES

Berman, L. (1988). Dilemmas in teaching caring: An "outsider's" perspective. *Scholarly Inquiry Into Nursing Practice, 1*(3), 1–14.

Bevis, E. O. (1988). New directions for a new age. In National League for Nursing (Ed.), *Curriculum revolution: Mandate for Change* (pp. 27–52). New York: National League for Nursing.

Bigge, M. L. (1982). *Educational philosophies for teachers.* Columbus: Merrill.

Buber, M. (1958). *I and thou* (Ronald G. Smith, Trans.). New York: Scribner.

Dewey, J. (1897). My pedagogic creed. *The School Journal, 54*(3), 77–80.

Freire, P. (1974). *Pedagogy of the oppressed* (Myra Bergman Ramos, Trans.). New York: Seabury Press.

Kaseworm, C. (1980). The older student as an undergraduate. *Adult Education, 31,* 30–37.

Knowles, M. (1973). *The adult learner: A neglected species.* Houston: Gulf Press.

LaMonica, E. L. (1985). *The humanistic nursing process.* Monterey, CA: Wadsworth.

McDaniels, O. B. (1983). Existentialism and pragmatism: The effect of philosophy on methodology of teaching. *Journal of Nursing Education, 22*(2), 62–68.

Morris, V. C. (1966). *Existentialism in education: What it means.* New York: Harper & Row.

Morris, V. C., & Pai, Y. (1976). *Philosophy and the American school.* Boston: Houghton-Mifflin.

National League for Nursing (Ed.). (1988). *Curriculum revolution: Mandate for change.* New York: National League for Nursing.

Osmon, H. A., & Craver, S. M. (1986). *Philosophical foundations of education.* Columbus: Merrill.

Reilly, D. E., & Oermann, M. H. (1985). *The clinical field: Its use in nursing education.* Norwalk, CT: Appleton-Century-Crofts.

Sakalys, J., & Watson, J. (1986). Professional education: Post-baccalaureate education for professional nursing. *Journal of Professional Nursing, 2*(3), 91–97.

Sarter, B. (1987). Evolutionary idealism: A philosophy for holistic nursing theory. *Advances in Nursing Science, 9*(2), 1–9.

Sartre, J. P. (1974). *Existentialism and human emotions.* New York: Philosophical Library.

Schon, D. (1987). *Educating the reflective practitioner: Toward a new design for teaching and learning in the professions.* San Francisco: Jossey-Bass.

Weintrout, M. (1983). Martin Buber: Philosopher of the I-thou dialogue. *Educational Theory, 13,* 50–57.

Weller, R. H. (1976). One perspective on humanistic education. In R. Weller (Ed.), *Humanism in education: Visions and realities.* Berkeley, CA: McCutchan.

Whitehead, A. N. (1967). *The aims of education and other essays.* Cambridge: Cambridge University Press.

Wineberg, C. (1972). *Humanistic foundations of education.* Englewood Cliffs, NJ: Prentice-Hall.

22

Creating a Caring Environment: Moral Obligations in the Role of Dean

Anne Boykin

Role may be defined as a position in an organizational structure, as the behaviors exhibited by the person in the position, or as the part a person plays. In 1981, the American Association of Colleges of Nursing (AACN) described the major dimensions of the dean's role as a person, a colleague, a scholar, and an administrator (Gallagher, 1988). The style in which these roles are lived reflects the philosophical orientation of the person. To create a caring environment, moral obligations and decision making inherent in the role of dean are directed from the premise that caring is the essence of nursing.

Roach (1987) affirms that caring as the human mode of being is a "presupposition for all activities designed to develop the capacity to care professionally" (p. 49). She stresses that an understanding of caring is integral to nursing and states that "without a focus on caring, reflections about nursing and their application to education, service, administration, and research would be analogous to spokes of a wheel deprived of both hub and rim—removed from focus, center, and identifiable boundaries" (1984, p. 4).

Roach identifies the ontical framework as one way to focus inquiry on caring. Onticology involves the study of an entity in its actual relation with other entities. Ontical questions include those which address obligations entailed in caring. Roach studied the functional and ethical

247

manifestations of caring through the question, What is a nurse doing when she (or he) is caring? These manifestations are referred to as the attributes of caring and include five *C*'s: compassion, competence, confidence, conscience, and commitment.

This chapter illustrates how Roach's five *C*'s provide a framework for reflection on self as a caring person and for creating a caring academic environment in the role of dean. The roles of dean as person and administrator will be discussed. Ideas presented are grounded phenomenologically in the author's five years of experience as director of a nursing program.

DEAN AS PERSON

Commitment

Commitment is defined by Roach as a "complex affective response characterized by a convergence between one's desires and one's obligations, and by a deliberate choice to act in accordance with them" (1989, p. 66). Commitment includes devotion. Mayeroff (1971) states, "devotion is essential to caring . . . when devotion breaks down, caring breaks down" (p. 8). Obligations arising from devotion are constituent elements in caring.

Personal commitments reflect our views as to the nature of being human and relationships. These commitments determine our way of being with self and others. If the ontological basis for living is that caring is the human mode of being and therefore to be human is to care, then I accept that I am a caring person and accept the obligations that rest with this. Moral obligations arise from our commitments. Therefore, when I make a commitment to caring as a way of being, I have become morally obligated.

Caring for self as a person requires courage to honestly know self and be responsive to the needs to grow. This process requires genuineness and openness. Active patience is needed to enlarge the living space resulting in freeing of self, to let go of the familiar and secure, and to create meaning for life. Loving and respecting self are essential to creating a caring environment.

Compassion

Roach describes compassion "as a way of living born out of an awareness of one's relationship to all living creatures; engendering a response of participation in the experience of another; a sensitivity to the pain and brokenness of the other; a quality of presence which allows one to share with and make room for the other" (1987, p. 58). According to Fox, "compassion operates at the same level as celebration because what is of most moment in compassion is not feelings of pity, but feelings of togetherness" (1979, p. 4). It is this union or togetherness that urges us to rejoice at another's joy (celebration) and to grieve at another's sorrow. Both these dimensions are integral to true compassion. Therefore, to develop compassion means to develop an awareness of the interdependence of all living things.

Compassion necessitates experiencing humaneness and knowing self so others may be better understood. There is a continuous consciousness of self and others as being caring and interconnected. I must learn to let go in order to remember the common base that unifies humankind.

Conscience

Conscience is a "state of moral awareness; a compass directing one's behavior according to the moral fitness of things" (Roach, 1987, p. 64). Conscience is an individual's way of tapping wisdom and insight within self and develops with experience and knowledge. Caring expresses itself in responsivity—responding to something that matters. Reflection on this thought should stimulate the asking of the question, Why ought the commitment be kept? It is the commitment that directs the "ought."

How ought a caring person be? There must be continual striving to experience self as other and yet be one with self, to be attuned to the values and the moral fitness of things, to value self in my own right and as unique and to develop greater ethical sensitivity or critical consciousness.

Competence

Competence, according to Roach (1987), is the "state of having the knowledge, judgment, skill, energy, experience and motivation required to respond adequately to the demands of one's professional responsibilities" (p. 61). On a personal level, one must become competent in caring.

Confidence

Confidence is the "quality which fosters trusting relationships" (Roach, 1987, p. 63). Confidence in caring promotes trust without dependency and portrays respect for self as person. As competence in caring develops, likewise does confidence.

DEAN AS ADMINISTRATOR

It is the person role that permeates each of the other roles of dean identified by AACN. Who and how I am as person influences who and how I am as colleague, scholar, and administrator. Therefore, the first moral obligation in the role of dean as administrator would be to be authentic to one's personhood. Concomitant with the moral obligations to self as person, the dean in the role of administrator assumes additional moral obligations. These obligations will be addressed using the framework of the five C's.

Commitment

Moral obligations in the role of dean include those relevant to self as person and as administrator. Decisions are made with caring as the moral basis for determining right action. How do actions of the dean reflect the moral commitment to caring? Obligations of dean include those to the profession and program, administration, faculty, students, the community, and society.

Obligations: Profession and Program.   The following questions provide a framework for reviewing obligations of the dean to the profession and program:

• To what am I committed?
• What content should a nursing program include and label nursing?
• If caring is the essence of nursing, how is it modeled in the role of dean so it is recognizable by others?
• How does the belief that caring is unique in nursing influence the design of the program?
• What are the obligations of the dean for guiding creative endeavors?
• What ought the administrative design of a caring-based program look like?

The following definition and goal of nursing directs the answers to some of these questions. Nursing is a "discipline of knowledge and field of professional practice which focuses on the human person patterning wellness. The goal of nursing is the promotion of the process of being and becoming through caring" (Faculty, Division of Nursing, Florida Atlantic University). Caring in nursing is understood as a uniquely human process in which the nurse artistically responds to a call from the client through authentic presence. With these beliefs in mind, the dean must create a freeing environment in which faculty can unlock the strong ties of the traditional past and explore the meaning of a caring-based nursing program. The commitment to caring as the essence of nursing necessitates a willingness to be influenced even when this requires entering into unknown territory. As Farley (1986) states, "only if we are open to new meanings for the past can we risk flexibility in our expectations of the future. Without this kind of flexibility, we cannot sustain hope. For unless we are open to new meaning in the future, there is no real future; there is only the past" (p. 57).

The model for the administrative design of a caring-based program is unfolding. It is envisioned that such a design would be analogous to Fox's (1979) description of "dancing Sarah's circle." The dancers in this model have a commitment to nursing in common. As these dancers form an open circle the incalculable worth of other is recognized and valued. Each dancer makes unique contributions to the program's unfolding. As administrator, the special and important administrative caring strategies and knowledges are brought to the circle. There is mutual interdependence and sharing. In a caring-based model, there is no room for contaminated competition but a love for being and creating together what ought to be.

Obligations: Administration. Visualizing top administrators as part of the open circle model is empowering. Administrators are not better than or more powerful than others in the circle. They, too, bring to the circle unique contributions that must be understood to appreciate their role and to influence the growth of caring in the overall system. As dean, the skill of using alternating rhythms to know others and to create caring moments is essential. The dean is obligated to help the system understand the goals of the nursing program and to secure the resources necessary to achieve its goals.

Obligations: Faculty. A major obligation of dean to faculty is to ground all actions in the commitment to caring. Devotion is evident in the worth placed in the other. The dean can create a freeing atmosphere where the becoming of faculty is encouraged and supported. Faculty are valued as colleagues and are not considered "my" faculty. Faculty are expected to negotiate teaching assignments with each other for they best know how they would like to grow. This freedom decreases territoriality and provides a greater opportunity to participate in the fullest sense. Time for scholarship and open dialogue is safeguarded.

Obligations: Students. The dean of a caring-based nursing program must model a way of being with students that portrays respect. The dean assists in creating an environment that fosters the development of the students' capacity to care. Informal dialogue between the dean and students on nursing offers an opportunity to share perceptions of the meaning and privilege of being a nurse. Caring is evident through authentic presence and openness. Policy formulation and implementation allow for unique student situations to be considered. During the educational process, there is an obligation to develop fully moral caring beings.

Obligations: Community/Society. The dean is in a position to act as liaison with the community. It is important to know from them their perceptions of nursing and their views on and commitment to the program. Nursing's unique role must be articulated and its value understood. Understanding the meaning of a caring-based nursing program by consumers of health care enhances commitment and facilitates the securing of resources needed to achieve program excellence.

Conscience in Caring

The dean of a caring-based program should ask the following question: How ought I to be as a caring administrator? In the role of administrator there are many decisions to be made. Decisions must be made with a commitment to caring. Therefore, conscience continually increases the commitment to caring as the moral fitness of decisions is examined. Within all aspects of administration, conscience promotes increased attention on the issues of values and beliefs. As my commitment moves to the future, I must choose again and again to ratify the commitment or not. Commitment to caring remains binding and the choices are based on devotion to this commitment.

Compassion in Caring

How is caring expressed in relationships inherent in the role of dean? Compassion, according to Fox, implies searching for authentic problems and workable solutions born of deeper and deeper questions (1979, p. 24). To understand the world of the other, opportunities for open, honest dialogue should be created. As the meaning of situations is better understood, creative and new solutions emerge. Through personal knowing of administrators, faculty and students, the dean is able to know the other's needs and desires and to imagine him or herself in the other's place. Choices therefore, are made with a lens that has considered all views. Mayeroff (1971) states, "when I help the other grow, I don't impose my own direction, but I allow the direction of the other as independent in its own right with needs that are to be respected" (p. 7).

Competence in Caring

Is my caring perceived by others? As an administrator of a caring-based program, I am obligated to become skilled in the use of the caring ingredients: knowing, alternating rhythms, trust, hope, courage, humility, patience, and honesty (Mayeroff, 1971). One example of essential knowing in this role is determination of budget. The budgetary process is critical to creating a caring environment. From a caring perspective, it must be the commitment that drives the budget rather than the budget that drives the commitment.

The complexities of human care assume the coexistence of competence and compassion. Roach (1987) states that competence without compassion is "brutal and inhumane" and compassion without competence is a "meaningless intrusion into the life of another" (p. 61).

Confidence in Caring

In what way has caring influenced my relationship? Confidence in caring is gained as commitments are tested. As results are seen, confidence and faith with caring grows.

SUMMARY

Mayeroff (1971) states "from a loose stringing together of ideas a tight fabric emerges; ideas intertwine and tend to reinforce each other, making for a mutual deepening of meaning and gain in precision" (p. 12). The fabric throughout this discussion is nursing. Commitment, compassion, confidence, competence, and conscience represent the ideas that, when uniquely and beautifully woven together, create the aesthetic experience of caring in nursing. The dean of a caring-based nursing

program is morally obligated to foster an environment that reflects a
commitment to caring.

REFERENCES

Farley, M. (1986). *Personal commitments: Making, keeping, breaking.* San Francisco:
    Harper & Row.

Fox, M. (1979). *Spirituality named compassion.* Minneapolis, MN: Winston Press.

Gallagher, R. M. (1988). The role of dean: A faculty perspective. *Nurse Educator,*
    13(2), 10–11.

Mayeroff, M. (1971). *On caring.* New York: Harper & Row.

Roach, S. (1984). *Caring: The human mode of being. Implications for nursing.*
    Toronto: Faculty of Nursing, University of Toronto, Perspectives in
    Caring, Monograph I.

Roach, S. (1987). *The human act of caring.* Ottawa: Canadian Hospital Association.

23

Caring as the Central Focus in Nursing Curriculum Development

Janet A. Bauer

Since the time of Nightingale, the terms *care* and *caring* have been consistently used in the nursing literature (Leininger, 1981). Nursing traditionally has been concerned with the caring needs of people and caring as a value or principle for guiding nursing action (Gaut, 1983).

Caring is said to be synonymous with nursing, inextricably linked to nursing, and the very heart of nursing (Griffin, 1983; Jordan, 1983; Wolf, 1986). Donnelly and Sutterley (1986) described caring as "the cornerstone of nursing" (p. vii). Current nursing literature describes caring as the essence and the central unifying, and dominant domain to characterize nursing (Benner & Wrubel, 1989; Leininger, 1984a, 1986; Watson, 1985). The American Nurses' Association (1980) stated, "nurses are guided by a humanistic philosophy having caring coupled with understanding and purpose as its central feature" (p. 18). Furthermore, Leininger stated:

> Although care is one of the most illusive and "taken for granted" concepts in nursing, it nevertheless remains the heart of nursing. It is what clients want most from nurses and the nursing profession (1986, p. 2).

255

While the nursing profession may subscribe to care and caring as dominant themes throughout its history, some nurses view these concepts as receiving limited emphasis in nursing practice and nursing education. According to Ray (1981), both individual and collective care has been receiving less and less emphasis in hospital and community health systems because of increased technological demands, emphasis on the medical model of cure, and economic competition within the health care industry.

Likewise, Watson (1985) stated that the human care role is threatened by increased medical technology and bureaucratic constraints in today's society. From observation, McWilliams (1976) concluded that few people have a hospital experience without feeling to some degree depersonalized and deprived of basic human rights and dignities. The increase in specialization and the development of science and technology has led to what Carper (1979) called an "erosion of care." As Naisbitt (1982) reported, when society is confronted with high technology, there must be a counterbalancing human response that is high-touch. For nursing this response is caring.

From a nursing education perspective, the teaching of care theories, concepts, and principles has received less emphasis than disease processes, body functioning, technologic procedures, and drug administration in most undergraduate and graduate nursing programs (Leininger, 1984b). In addition, most basic nursing textbooks and nursing dictionaries did not define the terms *care* or *caring*. Most references to the terms related to the notion "care of the person with . . . " or "nursing care of . . . ," and the concept of "nursing care plans" (Bauer, 1988). However, Watson (1985) stated,

> In order for nursing to be truly responsive to the needs of society and make contributions that are consistent with its roots and early origins, both nursing education and the health care delivery system must be based on human values and concern for the welfare of others. Caring outcomes in practice, research, and theory depend on the teaching of a caring ideology (p. 32).

Furthermore, if caring is a central component of professional nursing, as these discussions suggest, a pertinent question presented by Gaut (1984), Leininger (1984b), and MacDonald (1984) was, How is that concept being taught in nursing programs? Within the past decade, a few nursing programs have developed curricular frameworks based on the concept of caring. This chapter is based on a study investigating the teaching of caring in schools using such a framework (Bauer, 1988).

RESEARCH DESIGN

The purpose of this study was to ascertain the caring content and experiences included as components of selected baccalaureate nursing curricula. The study was conducted in three public college/university and two private/parochial schools of nursing located in the southern, midwestern, and western United States. A phenomenological design was used, with a convenience sample of 26 faculty and 32 senior nursing students. The five nursing programs were all National League for Nursing (NLN)-accredited, offered baccalaureate degrees, and used caring as a central theme in the program's conceptual framework. Data were collected from written curricular documents and personal open-ended group audiotaped interviews with the faculty members and students from each school. The interviews focused on descriptions of caring and how it was taught in the nursing curriculum. The findings of the study are presented as they relate to (1) the philosophy of caring in curricula, (2) caring content, (3) learning experiences, and (4) curricular outcomes.

PHILOSOPHY OF CARING IN CURRICULA

A nursing program philosophy is expected to be used as a guide for implementation of a curriculum. In accreditation materials, the National League for Nursing defines a philosophy as:

> a set of beliefs and value statements about the practice of nursing and the teaching of nursing, developed by the faculty, which provide direction for implementation of the curriculum (1983).

The curriculum for each school of nursing emerged from a philosophy and conceptual framework focusing on caring as a major concept or construct.

The philosophy for each school of nursing was based on either an existential humanistic or religious framework promoting the value, worth, dignity, and growth of human beings as the foundation for caring. Caring as an interpersonal process and the essence of nursing was also a component of the program philosophies and conceptual frameworks, which in turn provided the organization for each of the curricula. The entire curriculum was planned around caring. These philosophical beliefs directed the faculty in stating end of program objectives, developing and sequencing courses, course content selection, development of learning experiences, and approaches to teaching. As one student stated, "caring is the glue that holds the rest of the conceptual framework together."

CARING CONTENT

Caring content and learning experiences were organized to operationalize the philosophy and conceptual framework beginning with the first nursing course and continuing throughout the program of study. Course content presented caring as an interpersonal process central to and the very essence of nursing. A variety of traditional and nontraditional teaching methods and strategies were used to reflect the current state of knowledge about the concept of caring, attributes of caring, and the use of caring in nursing practice.

The term *caring content* reflected the phenomenon labeled as caring and its use as specific subject matter in the curriculum. Various philosophical teachings, including the writings of Mayeroff, religious writings, and writings of nurse theorists on caring, such as Bevis and Murray, Leininger, Watson, and others, formed a framework for presenting professional nursing content. Caring content was organized around the eight themes identified in Table 1.

Content Labeled as Caring

Content labeled as caring included the school's philosophy, conceptual framework, and program requirements; philosophical and theoretical

Table 1
Caring Content Themes

Content labeled as caring

Caring about self and others

Holistic care

Attributes of caring

Skills emphasizing caring component

Nursing process

Research on caring

Scope of nurse caring role

definitions of caring; components of the caring experiences, caring behaviors, and attributes; values, belief systems, and spiritual care; and traditional and nontraditional approaches to caring. Professional caring by
the nurse was emphasized as content and included developing a sound
knowledge base, nursing as a discipline of knowledge and professional
practice, components of professional caring, and caring as being the core
of nursing and touching every facet of nursing.

Caring about Self and Others

In learning to practice caring, one needs to learn to care about self
and others. Specific content on learning to care about self and others
focused on meeting one's physical, emotional, cognitive, social, and
spiritual needs. Developing self-awareness, techniques of stress management, and the development of support systems were emphasized.

Holistic Care

An holistic approach to client/patient care was another way of operationalizing the caring philosophy. Promoting the existential view of man
as having dignity, worth, value, and deserving of care was emphasized by
using an holistic approach to all aspects of care.

Attributes of Caring

Attributes of caring were terms identified as characteristics, qualities, or notions ascribed to being caring. Approximately 80 terms were
listed as attributes of caring. The goal of all attributes of caring was
promotion of growth in self or another individual. Allowing one to do
as he or she pleased, passing a student when he or she had not pro-
gressed satisfactorily, or doing everything for someone were identified
as being non-caring. These behaviors were not helpful in promoting
growth in another. Caring was said to be "tough love" and included
confrontation and limit setting, in addition to empathetic approaches to
individuals. The attributes of caring were taught as content in classes
and clinical practice.

Skills Emphasizing Caring Component

A variety of skills were taught as avenues for operationalizing caring.
Specific content using a caring framework focused on developing skill

with communication, interpersonal relationships, values clarification, technical and psychomotor skills, use of critical thinking, and the teaching and learning process. One school taught "hug therapy" as a way of physically demonstrating caring.

Nursing Process/Research on Caring/ Scope of Nurse Caring Role

The nursing process was taught as a systematic approach to the delivery of care and as the avenue for demonstrating professional caring. In addition, content on caring also reflected discussion of research relative to the concept. Research on caring was studied from the perspective of the nurse and the client. Lastly, content on the scope of the nurse caring role including the role of the professional nurse, professional role expectations, legal and ethical aspects of nursing, and the breadth of the nursing role were related to caring.

The eight themes emphasized the current state of knowledge about the concept of caring and became the framework for teaching nursing in these programs. The focus was on conveying information regarding philosophical notions, definitions, and theoretical perspectives of the concept; relating caring to college and nursing program requirements; development of a sound knowledge base, descriptions of attributes of caring, and the use of caring in nursing practice; analysis of caring notions throughout research and other literature; and incorporation of caring into one's personal and professional way of life.

CARING LEARNING EXPERIENCES

Caring experiences reflect learning activities used to facilitate mastery of caring content and how acquisition of knowledge of the phenomenon labeled as caring was achieved. Five major themes representing caring experiences appear in Table 2.

Organizational Plan for Caring in the Curriculum

The organizational plan for caring content and experiences throughout the program of study began with the initial course. Introducing caring concepts, including the school's philosophy and conceptual framework in the first nursing course, provided a foundation for the entire curriculum. Caring was a planned component of all major

Table 2
Learning Experiences Themes

Organizational plan for caring in the curriculum

Caring as a program expectation

Specific learning experiences reflecting caring

Strategies used to teach/learn caring

Role modeling in teaching caring

nursing courses with clinical assignments described as being specific learning experiences in caring.

Caring as a Program Expectation

Caring as a program expectation reflected anticipated student characteristics prior to entering nursing, desired attitudinal outcomes, ways of learning to treat clients in a caring manner, and ways of caring for one's self to avoid nurse burnout. Treating the mannequin as a person with respect and privacy was emphasized as a program expectation that "really teaches them" about caring. Caring was described as a way of life and as a part of nursing. Faculty and students stated that caring and nursing are not two separate things, but nursing is caring and all nursing behaviors are described as caring behaviors.

Specific Learning Experiences Reflecting Caring

Specific learning experiences reflecting caring included a variety of traditional and nontraditional learning activities. Clinical assignments provided an opportunity to practice and act out caring behaviors. The physical demonstration of caring behaviors was facilitated by two projects used by one school. These projects included providing "hug therapy" at a community wellness fair. Participants at the fair were given tickets to redeem for a hug. The hug therapy was directed at recognizing the value of giving and receiving physical contact as a way of helping people feel good. A second project was the giving of strokes or "warm fuzzies" (use of tokens) to tangibly recognize and reward caring behaviors identified in others. A strokes bazaar was a social activity for students, faculty, and staff to redeem the tokens for gift items.

Analysis of classic literature such as the *Parable of the Prince* and Dante's *Inferno* with identification of caring components and application to caring behaviors was another type of learning experience. An assignment to talk with geriatric clients about how they felt about their lives and aging and working in nursing homes with elderly clients were additional specific learning experiences aimed at learning caring.

Strategies Used to Teach/Learn Caring

Various strategies used to teach/learn caring were identified, including such traditional teaching methods as lecture and discussions; post-conferences and seminars; small group exercises and activities involving case studies, role-play situations, critical analysis techniques; films and videotapes of situations; testing over caring content; and clinical evaluation of caring behaviors. Giving strokes and the strokes bazaar was another strategy used for teaching caring.

Faculty behaviors were also identified as major strategies for teaching caring, for example:

1. Instilling feelings of self-worth in students.
2. Being available, willing to become involved with students and spending time with them.
3. Stating performance expectations and setting limits.
4. Sensitivity to student needs.
5. Providing both positive and negative feedback.
6. Providing encouragement and support.
7. Demonstrating a prevailing belief that one cannot teach caring if one really doesn't display it.

Role Modeling in Teaching Caring

Role modeling of caring was also identified as having an impact on students' learning caring. In this study, faculty role modeling was identified by both faculty members and students as the most important way faculty teach caring. Faculty role model through demonstration of caring with clients, students, and other faculty; assisting students in clinical situations and with personal struggles; and providing examples to students of how to deal with varying situations. Congruence between what faculty say and demonstrate by role modeling in the clinical area was said to have a major effect on nursing students learning caring. A student quote aptly summarizes this notion:

> Faculty always do the things that we've been taught to do. . . . PhD instructor doing what you've been taught to do and treating every human being with dignity. . . . If it was wiping a bottom or giving an injection, same dignity. . . . Every job has dignity when it's done with caring. . . . That's been a nonverbal experience to me from all the instructors I've ever had in clinical in this school . . . and that has impressed me.

Students' role modeling caring was another way of learning about this concept. Observing the skills of other students in class, in the clinical areas, and during social and other contact served as an avenue for learning caring. In addition, nursing staff provided both positive and negative role models for caring and were learning experiences for students. Negative role modeling by nursing staff was discussed and analyzed in post-conferences, and alternative ways of behaving in various situations were generated.

A further role model for caring was the school's director or administrator. Caring was said to start with the department head and filter throughout the program. An open-door policy by the director reflected an availability to faculty and students and a model of caring.

Last, one school stated the example of Jesus as providing a model for caring. The use of Biblical passages gave insight into behaviors Jesus demonstrated as acts of caring and were applied to nursing care situations.

Learning experiences promote active involvement with the concept of caring for acquisition of knowledge. Clinical experiences and other experiential activities provide opportunities for application and practice of caring concepts. Identifying with role models exemplifying caring is a major way students learn caring. Faculty role modeling—by demonstrating a congruence between what is presented as content and the use of those caring behaviors when dealing with clients, students, and other faculty—is a key to effectively teaching caring.

ANTICIPATED CURRICULAR OUTCOMES

This study suggested various anticipated outcomes of using the attributes of caring and the impact of emphasizing caring in the curriculum. Outcomes identified from teaching caring included:

1. The nurse feeling a sense of satisfaction and reward, increased motivation with decreased competition, increased understanding of one's self and others, and development of interpersonal relationships.
2. Clients/patients feeling better as a result of caring behaviors.
3. Caring behaviors promoting reciprocal reactions between the client/patient and the nurse.
4. Students internalizing caring values and transferring these behaviors into practice settings.

Furthermore, caring was said to be physically and emotionally exhausting and may result in burnout if one gives too much of the self without meeting one's personal needs.

SUMMARY

Nursing literature and conferences are advocating a return to the humanistic values and caring approach to people that has been a hallmark of nursing. A theory base for caring in nursing is emerging. Over the past 10 years several research studies in nursing have focused on the concept of caring. Most studies have dealt with defining and understanding the concept of caring and identifying attributes of caring from the perspective of the patient/client and from that of the nurse.

New work on caring is looking at teaching of the concept in schools of nursing (Bauer, 1988), the economics of caring (Buerhaus, 1986), the relationship between caring and nurse burnout (Gustafson, 1984), issues of ethics and caring (Fry, 1988 & 1989), to name just a few. The concept of caring is being legitimized as an area appropriate for nurses to study.

As nursing educators know, building a program on a strong philosophical base with faculty committed to implementation of the program philosophy is crucial for success of program outcome. Using a caring framework for teaching nursing exposes nursing students to more than an empirical basis for practice. An holistic approach to really understanding people as human beings of value, worth, and having needs becomes the focus of content.

To effectively teach caring, faculty must role model the attributes of caring to nursing students. This involves accepting and treating students as having value, worth, and the potential for growth. Faculty must also feel good about themselves and their abilities as teachers. Faculty need to feel confident and comfortable in their role as educators, master their subject matter, and be willing to get involved with students. Faculty development programs, recruitment of faculty espousing a caring philosophy, and mentoring new faculty into their modeling role are important considerations for the effective teaching of caring.

Promoting a caring framework for nursing and faculty modeling of caring behaviors and attitudes could affect student recruitment. In our highly technologic society, great emphasis is being placed on person-to-person relationships. Reaffirming the caring nature of nursing to the public and actively promoting these behaviors may make the nursing profession a more attractive and appealing career choice.

REFERENCES

Bauer, J. A. (1988). Caring content and experiences as components of baccalaureate nursing curricula: A phenomenological study. *Dissertation Abstracts International.* (University Microfilms 88-16, 392)

Benner, P., & Wrubel, J. (1989). *The primacy of caring: Stress and coping in health and illness.* Menlo Park, CA: Addison-Wesley.

Buerhaus, R. I. (1986). The economics of caring: Challenges and new opportunities for nursing. *Topics in Clinical Nursing, 8*(2), 13–21.

Carper, B. A. (1979). The ethics of caring. *Advances in Nursing Science, 1*(3), 11–19.

Criteria for the evaluation of baccalaureate and higher degree programs in nursing. (1983). New York: National League for Nursing.

Donnelly, G. F., & Sutterley, D. C. (1986). From the editors. *Topics in Clinical Nursing, 8*(2), vii.

Fry, S. (1988). The ethic of caring: Can it survive in nursing? *Nursing Outlook, 36*(1), 48.

Fry, S. (1989). Toward a theory of nursing ethics. *Advances in Nursing Science, 11*(4), 9–21.

Gaut, D. A. (1983). Development of a theoretically adequate description of caring. *Western Journal of Nursing Research, 5*, 313–324.

Gaut, D. A. (1984). A theoretic description of caring. In M. M. Leininger (Ed.), *Care: The essence of nursing and health* (pp. 27–44). Thorofare, NJ: Slack.

Griffin, A. P. (1983). A philosophical analysis of caring in nursing. *Journal of Advanced Nursing, 8*, 289–295.

Gustafson, W. (1984). Motivational and historical aspects of care and nursing. In M. M. Leininger (Ed.), *Care: The essence of nursing and health* (pp. 61–73). Thorofare, NJ: Slack.

Jordan, C. H. (1983). Caring and sharing: Spectrums of practice. *AORN JOUR-NAL, 38,* 1003–1007, 1010.

Leininger, M. M. (1981). The phenomenon of caring: Importance, research questions and theoretical considerations. In M. M. Leininger (Ed.), *Caring: An essential human need* (pp. 3–15). Thorofare, NJ: Slack.

Leininger, M. M. (1984a). Care: The essence of nursing and health. In M. M. Leininger (Ed.), *Care: The essence of nursing and health* (pp. 3–15). Thorofare, NJ: Slack.

Leininger, M. M. (1984b). Caring is nursing: Understanding the meaning, importance, and issues. In M. M. Leininger (Ed.), *Care: The essence of nursing and health* (pp. 83–93). Thorofare, NJ: Slack.

Leininger, M. M. (1986). Care facilitation and resistance factors in the culture of nursing. *Topics in Clinical Nursing, 8*(2), 1–11.

MacDonald, M. (1984). Caring—The central construct for an associate degree nursing curriculum. In M. M. Leininger (Ed.), *Care: The essence of nursing and health* (pp. 233–248). Thorofare, NJ: Slack.

McWilliams, R. M. (1976). The balance of caring. *AORN Journal, 24,* 314–317, 320–323.

Naisbitt, J. (1982). *Megatrends: Ten new directions transforming our lives.* New York: Warner.

Nursing: A social policy statement. (1980). Kansas City, MO: American Nurses' Association.

Ray, M. A. (1981). A philosophical analysis of caring within nursing. In M. M. Leininger (Ed.), *Caring: An essential human need* (pp. 25–36). Thorofare, NJ: Slack.

Watson, J. (1985). *Nursing: Human science and human care. A theory of nursing.* Norwalk, CT: Appleton-Century-Crofts.

Wolf, Z. R. (1986). Forward. *Topics in Clinical Nursing, 8*(2), viii.

24

Phenomenology of Self: An Experiential Approach to the Teaching and Learning of Caring

Linda J. Postlethwaite

This chapter addresses the question of how caring can be developed in nursing educationally. Presented are methods for study of "self" that provide direction in the educational development and integration of caring skills in nursing practice. As nurses are facilitated in educational settings to experience and express their personal knowing of self in caring relationship with others, their conscious repertoire of caring skills for practice is expanded and developed.

Nursing literature is replete with discussions of the meaning and place of caring in nursing, and with studies of the nature of caring in practice. Roach (1984) notes that the "personal, humanistic, spiritual motivation" (p. 42) that is the very basis of nursing is endangered. She challenges nursing to develop and empower the capacity of caring. Yet, little is available on how caring capacity may be enriched and how caring skills may be developed.

Caring is a lived experience, a personal inner knowing developed in and through one's ways of being in the world. Caring is expressed and experienced transpersonally—that is, in relation to others within the environment. Carper (1978) proposes that in order for nursing knowledge to be whole, personal knowing, which along with aesthetic knowing forms the foundation of the art of nursing, must be included. Carper acknowledges that these fluid dimensions of caring may be difficult to master and teach, but holds that it is "necessary for achieving mastery in the discipline" (pp. 21–22), that nursing find ways of doing so.

In this light, it is proposed that the self is a laboratory for awareness of the personal knowing of caring. The world is both teacher and classroom and the self is both teacher and student of caring. This paper presents in journal form one nurse's self-study in relation to caring. It describes components of the phenomenological process through which this nurse expanded her understanding and expression of self as a caring human being, and describes the integration of this personal knowing into her professional nursing practice. Specific experiential methods for the development of the personal knowing of caring in nursing are described. The example of this nurse's self-study provides direction for the development of personal, aesthetic, experiential content as a component of caring curricula. The train of thought leading to this quest in the personal knowing of self as caring began in a graduate nursing course, "Caring: Advanced Foundation of Nursing." That this is so is a testimony to the value of placing caring at the center of nursing curricula.

THE QUEST

Since teaching and learning are among the greatest joys in my life, during the caring course in my MSN program I avidly combed the literature to explore how the lived experience of caring is learned, and how the learning of caring is lived. While the literature contains much information on the concept and nature of caring, I did not find the answer to these questions. I chose to embark on a personal journey, to look at my self and my own development as a caring person and a nurse, to see if through personal knowing I could discover my own answers. The metaphor of a plant unfolding through the stages of germination, incubation, sprouting, growth, budding, blossoming, and bearing fruit provides a framework for the journal reflection of the unfolding of caring through my life experiences. And so, to begin, I go back to the beginning.

GERMINATION

At the age of 12, I spent a summer volunteering as a candy striper at a local hospital. I spent my time in a storage closet compiling chart forms into charts and was overjoyed when I was moved to a position in the coffee shop. It was a delight to be with people, and I felt that I was at last able to serve, even if only tuna fish sandwiches and milk shakes.

At the age of 14, I got my working papers and took my first paying job as a nurse's aid in a convalescent home. Reflecting on this decision and what led me to it, I would have to say it was an intuitive action. Truthfully, I have no remembrance of engaging in a conscious decision-making process about what kind of work I wanted to do. It never occurred to me to pursue checking groceries or working in a soda shop after school. A friend mentioned the job in the convalescent home and I knew that it was the right thing for me to do. I am not aware of any conscious altruistic motivation in choosing this work; it was as though, unbeknownst to me, a calling was moving me and I did not question it.

What I am aware of having learned in this role is the emptiness and loneliness of many old people at the end of their lives. I saw the glimmer of life it brought them to have someone touch them with love, to have youth and laughter in their space, to have someone dwell with them gently.

At the age of 16 during the late 1960s, social interest was awakening in me. I was conscious of wanting to serve people and felt courageous and strong in this cause. Again serendipity led me, this time to a home for abandoned, neglected, emotionally disturbed children. It was persistence that won me a position as a child care worker in a dormitory of 14 girls, 13 black and 1 caucasian, between the ages of 7 and 12. I experienced in this role the bitterness and anger that expressed the crystallized sadness, loneliness, and fear that exists in many young hearts that have seemingly not been touched by caring. Now I knew that it was not just our old folks that needed care but many young folks as well.

Still, my calling to help did not yet take focus and direction. I spent some time in transition from high school to college, from home to the world, and wondered what I might be when I grew up. My first college experiences were in Washington, DC, during the height of the peace protests against the Vietnam war. I listened to the Beatles and marched for peace and knew I wasn't ready to choose a career path. This being the case, I dropped out of college and moved to a rural area to live simply and learn who I was.

As I came into adulthood, I found myself again pursuing work in human service. This time I worked as a child care aide in the hospital of a state institution for the retarded. I cared for profoundly retarded children from ages 2 to 16. Here, I learned the common humanity of us all. I learned the peace and love we can bring through caring to even those we judge incapable of thinking, functioning and relating. I learned I wanted to be a nurse. At this point, I became aware of the seed of caring germinating within me.

INCUBATION

I supported myself through my early student nursing period working as a nurse's aid on an opthalmology unit in an acute-care hospital in New York City. In this position, I learned what it meant for people to feel they weren't whole and to have dependency imposed on them by their health situation.

Interestingly, my time in the associate degree nursing program seemed to have a flatness to it that belied the multidimensional human experiences that had led me to choose nursing. I took pride in my academic achievement and learned to know myself as a competent, technical nurse and grew in the empirical and ethical knowing of myself and of my new role of caregiving as a nurse. The flatness continued through my first position as an RN on a surgical floor of a large medical center in New York City. In retrospect, I see that the caring seed ready to sprout within me became encapsulated and went into incubation as I focused on technical, task-oriented skills and pathology.

SPROUTING AND UNFOLDING

Feeling incomplete and unfulfilled by my nursing work, I concluded that I must not know enough and went back to school for my BSN. It was my good fortune to select a school that reawakened and nurtured the caring seed within me. I was intuitively led once again, this time into exploration of both the science and art of nursing through the opportunity to study Martha Rogers' (1970) theoretical framework for nursing as part of my nursing theories coursework. I became inspired and challenged and felt I had found the missing link in my nursing practice as I explored the Rogerian world view. The ground it provided was fertile for growth into actualization of my caring capacity.

GROWTH

During the ensuing period, two factors fertilized my growth. The first was a position I held as a staff nurse in the newborn nursery while I worked my way through the baccalaureate program. This experience had a twofold impact on me. First, I was awed by the spiritual wonder of new life coming into being in the world, and the privileged, holistic role nurses potentially play in welcoming and facilitating the integration of their coming. Second, I was appalled by the apparent lack of sensitivity to this wonder and privilege I observed in my nursing peers. I left this position when it became clear that I was not able to instigate change. I was also motivated to learn all that I could about how to serve in a truly caring way. I went on to take a position as a clinical instructor in obstetrical nursing at a local associate degree program in nursing, which allowed me to support future nurses in exploring the issues, dilemmas, joys, and gifts of nursing in this area.

The other factor that supported my growth at this time was my introduction in my BSN program to therapeutic touch, a caring method and way of being based on skilled energy exchange between a caregiver and the one cared for. Developed by Dr. Dolores Krieger, a professor of nursing at New York University, it is grounded in the Rogerian framework and provides a direct path to the heart of nursing. I embraced the study and practice of therapeutic touch wholeheartedly and vowed never again to falter into unconsciousness about the true energetic nature of what transpires in the process of caring.

Three guidelines that I integrated from Krieger's work (1979) as prerequisites to the effective practice of therapeutic touch also became guidelines for me in keeping my vow. They are the processes of attending to motivation, centering, and intention. In brief, attending to motivation is not only a retrospective knowing of why one makes the choices one does in life—for example, why one chose to become a nurse. Rather, it involves exploring the ongoing choices one makes moment by moment in life. Why do I choose to be a nurse, in this moment? Why do I choose to help and heal others, in this moment? Where does my motivation lie in this action I am taking, in this moment?

Attending to centering is a choice to engage in self-discipline to gain skill in quieting and focusing one's self in order to be truly present to others in their service. Centering is essential to know and facilitate the energetic level of transpersonal relating that occurs between nurse and client in what Watson (1988) calls "the caring occasion" (p. 59). Attending to intention involves consciously choosing the quality and amount of energy being exchanged in each therapeutic interaction.

BUDDING AND BLOSSOMING

As I completed my BSN, I continued in a parallel process of study of therapeutic touch and became interested in extending it beyond my personal practice. I began to share therapeutic touch with other nurses through continuing education courses in our community.

My career in nursing entered an expansive stage when I accepted a position to design, implement and manage a holistic, inpatient-outpatient, interdisciplinary pain management center at a local hospital. I gathered a team of credentialled health care practitioners who were versed in the art and science of their disciplines and prepared to offer traditional and nontraditional approaches to clients. As a team, we based our philosophy on the Rogerian world view as a guide to holistic practice. I had a wonderful role that cut across all nursing practice areas—administration, education, and clinical practice. Therapeutic touch was integrated into the program and evolved to meet our clients' needs in new and creative ways, with excellent results.

At the same time that this professional budding was taking place, I experienced personal blossoming. Through my work, I had the opportunity to participate in a personal growth seminar, loving relationships training. In this training, participants explore their personal histories, the conscious and unconscious patterns established and lived in their lives, and methods to consciously direct personal, creative energies toward self-actualizing choices in all relationships, starting with the relationship with self. Initially, I embraced these relationship technologies and lifestyle management approaches on a personal level. In my next phase, I bridged over to bring them to bear on my professional role as a nurse.

BEARING FRUIT

This most recent phase is one in which I am bringing to fruition the full measure of caring I have cultivated. Entrance into a MSN program provided the transitional energy and reflective opportunity required. The course on caring stimulated the self-exploration that allowed me to discover the unity of meaning of all that had gone before. Beginning a scholarly review of caring, evolutionary idealism, consciousness, creativity, and patterning facilitated my process.

I am presently moved to develop ways for others to engage in this process of self-study. Combining a variety of consciousness-raising activities, insight approaches, and personal growth methodologies, I endeavor to support others to enter into their own process of personal knowing of self and caring.

To advance this process, I have designed a three-hour experiential self-study workshop. This workshop has been offered once, to a group of supervisory-level nurses at one acute-care hospital in the southeastern United States. A phenomenological study of the meaning of this workshop to the nurses that participated in it is in progress. The information emerging from this study should help to fill the gap in nursing knowledge between the knowing of the nature of caring in nursing and the knowing of the lived experience of learning caring.

The self-study workshop activities include self-awareness exercises, guided meditation, a written journal reflective of the participant's life experiences and patterns, and guided interpersonal sharing in pairs or small groups. The content addresses the participant's developmental and present experience of caring; modes of giving and receiving caring; attention to motivation, centering, and intention as potential guides to effectiveness in caring as a nurse; and patterns of creating caring, fun, and fulfillment in nursing. This workshop initiates an exploration of how one's personal values, feelings, thoughts, behaviors, and attitudes express the self in personal and professional ways.

REVIEW OF THE LITERATURE

The following is an abbreviated version of the review of the literature for the phenomenological study in progress. As Watson (1988b) states, "Nursing within a transpersonal perspective attends to the human center of both the one caring and the one cared for" (p. 177). It would seem that to live the meaning of those words fully, nurses must enter with open hearts and open minds into the study of self. For as Mayeroff (1971) has identified, "only because I understand and respond to my own needs to grow can I understand his [the other's] striving to grow; I can understand in another only what I can understand in myself" (p. 42).

The choice to review one's personal history as a starting point in this process may be supported by Watson (1979) when she indicates that humanistic values and altruistic behavior can be developed through consciousness raising and close examination of one's views, beliefs, and values, early experiences that aroused compassion and emotions, exposure to different cultures, and personal growth experiences.

Evidence is apparent in the literature that new, experiential approaches to the teaching and learning of caring are needed. Watson (1985) stated, "One reason that teaching is inadequate or ineffective in nursing is that the focus is on the teaching, rather than the interpersonal and learning components of the process" (p. 74). Though she was addressing patient teaching, this statement may be construed to have relevance to the pedagogy of nursing. Ray (1985) would seem to concur when she states,

> Although nursing has made some inroads into the study of caring, the objective and cognitive components tend to be examined rather than the equally important internal (intersubjective) structures of caring, which are essential attributes for clinical nurses to know (p. 85).

Benner and Wrubel (1989) discuss a variety of approaches that they feel to be useful in the patient teaching work nurses do which may also have relevance for nursing education. These include consciousness raising, insight therapy, and other personal growth methods, such as meditation.

In summary even this limited review of the literature acknowledges the gap in nursing knowledge between what caring is and how the learning of caring is lived in practice. Several authors (Carper, 1978; Bevis, 1981; Ray, 1985; Watson, 1985, 1988a) have written of the importance of personal knowing of self and caring in nursing. Methods for achieving this knowing that are congruent with those presented in this chapter may be gleaned and synthesized from nursing literature.

So that the experiential approaches discussed here may live for you as you traverse your own path to self-actualization through the learning and living of caring, several self-study exercises are presented here. While these processes may be done as individual written reflective processes, it is suggested that they are useful and have a different impact when shared as verbal processes with another, such as a nursing colleague.

Complete the following open-ended sentences:

Caring is . . .

A way I experienced caring while I was growing up is . . .

Other ways I experienced caring while I was growing up are . . .

Some ways I experience caring in my work are . . .

Some ways I express caring in my work are . . .

My motivation in being a nurse is . . .

Some negative thoughts I have about my work are . . .

My most negative thought about my work is . . .

What I envision as being my ideal work scene . . .

One month from now is . . .

Six months from now is . . .

What I envision as being my ideal work scene . . .

Two years from now is . . .

Ten years from now is . . .

One hundred years from now is . . .

Journalling: Using the metaphorical framework of the plant—germinating, incubating, sprouting and unfolding, growing, budding, blossoming, and bearing fruit—perhaps you will choose to trace and acknowledge the unfolding of caring in your life.

REFERENCES

Benner, P., & Wrubel, J. (1989). *The primacy of caring: Stress and coping in health and illness.* Menlo Park, CA: Addison-Wesley.

Bevis, E. O. (1981). Caring: A life force. In M. M. Leininger (Ed.), *Caring: An essential human need* (pp. 49–59). Thorofare, NJ: Slack.

Carper, B. A. (1978). Fundamental patterns of knowing in nursing. *Advances in Nursing Science,* 13–23.

Chamberlain, D. (1988). *Babies remember birth.* New York: Jeremy P. Tarcher.

Leininger, M. M. (July 1986). Care facilitation and resistance factors in the culture of nursing. *Topics in Clinical Nursing, 8*(2), 1–12.

Mayeroff, M. (1971). *On caring.* New York: Harper & Row.

Ray, M. A. (1981). A philosophical analysis of caring within nursing. In M. M. Leininger (Ed.), *Caring: An essential human need* (pp. 25–36). Thorofare, NJ: Slack.

Ray, M. A. (1985). A philosophical method to study nursing phenomena. In M. M. Leininger (Ed.), *Qualitative research methods in nursing.* New York: Greene & Stratton.

Roach, M. S. (1984). *Caring: The human mode of being. Implications for nursing.* Toronto: Faculty of Nursing, University of Toronto, Perspectives in Caring, Monograph I.

Rogers, M. E. (1970). *An introduction to the theoretical basis of nursing.* Philadelphia: F. A. Davis.

Watson, J. (1985). *The philosophy and science of caring.* Boston: Little, Brown.

Watson, J. (1988a). *Nursing: Human science and human care. A theory of nursing.* New York: National League for Nursing.

Watson, J. (November 1988b). New dimensions of human caring theory. *Nursing Science Quarterly, 1*(4), 175–181.

25

Learning Caring Behavior in an Integrated Manner

Diana Gendron

Should caring behavior be taught as a series or set of individual actions, or as integrated behavior? The position taken here is that learning caring actions as separate pieces of behavior (e.g., smiling or headnods) can result in awkward and self-conscious behavior in the caregiver. The neurological perspective of integrated behavior presented here reveals that patterns formed from experiencing caring situations and having values and goals of caring organize psychological and physiological processes that result in integrated caring actions. The chapter also identifies educational approaches that facilitate learning skilled actions. In addition, questions are raised about other learning approaches that could be further explored to promote the development of caring behaviors in an integrated manner.

AWARENESS AND INTEGRATED BEHAVIOR

Someone once asked the cartoon cat Garfield whether, when he walked, his right and left legs moved together or opposite each other. Somewhat puzzled, Garfield looked at his feet and thought about the question. He then concluded to himself that he would never walk again.

Walking, like so many other behaviors, is an integrated, coordinated activity that occurs without conscious awareness of each movement. In fact, conscious awareness can interrupt smooth, integrated actions. Pribram (1971) discussed the inverse relationship between awareness and behavior. When a person experiences the same situation repeatedly, the person habituates, that is, does not notice the repetitive events. Even though awareness decreases, performance ability increases. With a change in the situation, the person has an orienting response, that is, becomes aware. But this awareness has one limited ability to integrate performance (Bobrow & Norman, 1975; Hart, 1975; Pribram, 1971).

Caring has been described as an interpersonal art in which the matching and synchronizing of one's behavior with another person's needs is frequently rapid, with the specific dynamics of behavioral shifts usually below the caregiver's level of consciousness (Gendron, 1988). All the ways we communicate, for example, words, listening, body movement, touch, and use of space, can be described as being enacted in an integrated, context-sensitive manner. Specific behaviors, such as looking at the other person, leaning forward, and using touch, may be *observed* in looking at caring behavior. But a conscious focus on *doing* each of these actions overlooks the integrative characteristic of caring behavior.

VALUE OF A NEUROLOGICAL PERSPECTIVE

Benner (1984) and Benner and Wrubel (1988) have highlighted the need to give recognition to skilled action, or "know how," in nursing and in general behavior. They discuss skilled action from a phenomenological perspective, using terminology such as "the habitual body" (p. 71). Although this phenomenological perspective contributes a needed emphasis on the nonreflective immediacy of actions, it does not assist in understanding the underlying basis of skilled activity. The terminology of the perspective appears to illustrate Flannery and Taylor's (1981) observation of the sometimes mysterious leap from mind to body: "It seems . . . that what was being leaped over was the brain . . . " (p. 22).

Benner and Wrubel (1988) do include some discussion related to the role of the central nervous system in skilled behavior, and this chapter explores this role somewhat more. Skilled behavior is discussed from the perspectives of neurophysiology and neuropsychology; some of these ideas are then related to learning theory. Information from these perspectives support such major emphases of Benner and Wrubel as tacit knowledge and the importance of context. A neurological perspective will assist in linking ideas from a number of fields, thereby fostering model building and the development of educational approaches toward facilitating integrated caring behavior.

ASSOCIATION NETWORKS AND SCHEMATA

According to Hart (1983), there is strong evidence in the literature that, with our brains, we receive sensations from our experiences in a "multipath, multimodal" way (p. 55). In other words, there are many parallel mental processes occurring simultaneously (Gazzaniga, 1985; Hart, 1983; Pribram, 1980). Again according to Hart, our brain primarily detects *patterns* in our multiple perceptions and acts as the "integrative center for the nervous system" (p. 34).

Our previous experiences and learning are retained as patterns of information and sequences of action. These patterns are widely distributed in the brain as networks or webs of associated facts and events (John, 1980; Pribram, 1971). The various aspects of an experience and its context are interrelated. Pribram (1971) uses the analogy of the hologram and states, "Whether something is remembered is in large part a function of the form and context in which it is experienced" (p. 66). Because of the association networks of perceptions and memories, one aspect of an experience can elicit other aspects through these association networks. John (1980) has stated that "the anatomically extensive neural ensembles representing a whole memory can be activated by sight, sound, smells, moods, needs or movements that occurred during the earlier experience" (p. 101). Therefore, in nursing situations, learned caring actions are most naturally linked as association networks in the brain. Via these association networks, even subtle perceptions by the caregiver about the context and patient's behavior can elicit a holistic, nonreflective response by the caregiver.

A neurologically integrated pattern of expectations and responses is formed from past caring situations. These patterns are "inner contexts" or schemata that then influence how new information or experience is interpreted and how actions are performed. In the psychological literature Rumelhart (1980) describes the power of schemata. People who have difficulty interpreting a set of facts when an unfamiliar situation is described interpret the same facts with ease when a familiar situation is described. Having an inner context or schema makes the difference.

Thus we can speak of caring schemata. It is these schemata or caring patterns that need to be fostered in nursing education, not sets of isolated actions.

A HIGH-LEVEL PURPOSE
EVOKES INTEGRATED BEHAVIOR

We have hierarchies of neural ensembles and schemata that function in our brain (Bobrow & Norman, 1975; Gallwey, 1974; Hart, 1983; Pribram, 1971). A broad aim or intention, or a high-level purpose, can automatically evoke and entrain other ensembles of integrated actions. Gallwey (1974) provides a good example of this process in his book, *The Inner Game of Tennis.* An aim to throw up a ball and hit it with the middle of the racquet automatically coordinates simultaneous movements of posture and action that would be difficult to achieve by consciously focusing on exactly how to place arms, body, and legs and move each in sequence.

In terms of kinesthetic movements, Pribram (1971) discusses what he calls an "Image-of-Achievement" (p. 243) in the motor area of the cerebral cortex. This image-of-achievement is formed before acting and then coordinates actions via interrelationships with the basal ganglia, the cerebellum, and sensory receptors in muscles. An image-of-achievement enables an act to be accomplished by a variety of different muscular movements, not just one. The image does not move specific muscles, but senses degrees of force that muscles must exert to achieve the action. According to Pribram, "The model that emerges differs considerably from the conception of the motor cortex as a keyboard upon which the activities of the rest of the brain (and/or mind) converge to play a melody of movement. Rather, patterns of know-*how* here become encoded and make possible effective acts, the external representations of brain processes" (p. 250).

Caring behavior involves caring values and goals in concert with integrated kinesthetic actions. Pribram (1971) describes caring as context-sensitive behavior: "Caring for someone is not so much doing something as doing it at the right time in the right place, when needs are felt and communicated" (p. 351). He identifies the fronto-limbic system of the brain as crucial to rapid monitoring and adjustment of behavior. An internal pragmatic context is established by the fronto-limbic system so that our highest level of aims and values are used to gauge ongoing experiences and stimulate appropriate actions organized by the motor areas of the brain. The intention to care can thus itself evoke integrated caring behaviors. Can we develop more approaches that would encourage learners to think about caring and vividly imagine what their caring might feel and look like? Can we also evoke integrated caring behavior by finding ways to stimulate in learners a pragmatic context of concern for and interest in others?

The intention to care can be viewed as somewhat analogous to an image-of-achievement in that it is an aim that can neurologically organize integrated behavior. Another way of describing an aim that can organize integrated expression is Suzanne Langer's concept of an "idea" or "imagined form" (in Gendron, 1988, pp. 29, 30) which functions as a broad aim that guides artistic creation. When caring was discussed as an art, a basic pattern of the multidimensional aspects of caring behavior was described by Gendron as "union and separation toward growth" (p. 29). The caregiver may, therefore, use the concept of union and separation toward growth as an imagined form, or what could be called a pragmatic context, that could guide caring behavior in a dynamic, fluid and integrated way.

DECLARATIVE AND PROCEDURAL KNOWLEDGE

Investigators of memory describe types of knowledge as declarative or procedural (Cohen & Squire, 1980; Pribram, 1971; Squire, 1984). Just as Benner (1984) has used the distinctions "know that," or declarative knowledge, and "know how," or procedural knowledge, these terms are being used to describe what seem to be two memory systems that we have. Studies show that learning can occur without recall, or declarative knowledge, and sometimes without awareness. In fact, the difference between the two memory systems may be awareness.

Several studies show that amnesic patients can learn procedural knowledge, for example, perceptual-motor and problem-solving skills, even though they do not remember the learning sessions (Cohen & Squire, 1980; Squire, 1984). People without memory deficits perform better on certain word tests after previous exposure to the words even though they do not remember seeing the words before (Schacter & Moscovitch, 1984). Studies of people who have had their corpus callosums split, or so-called "split-brain" patients, can respond appropriately to certain pictures, but are not aware that they have seen the pictures (Gazzaniga, 1985). All of these studies point toward conscious awareness as one ability of our brain, but in many instances only as a small part of its functioning. *We* are far more than our conscious awareness. The recognition that procedural knowledge can occur without awareness implies that learners of caring behavior can acquire integrated "know how" in ways that do not specifically call their attention to the behaviors.

LEARNING APPROACHES

Learned, integrated behavior can readily be transferred to a new situation if the new situation has a pattern similar to previous situations in which the integrated behavior was used (Hart, 1983). One educator, Leslie Hart, has developed a theory of learning in which he uses many characteristics of brain functioning, including the concept of a hierarchy of processes and the transfer of abilities to similar situations. Can we not assume that learners of professional caring behavior have used many aspects of integrated caring actions before, for example, with friends and family members, or with pets or a plant? Are there ways we can better link professional learning to these already acquired, integrated caring behaviors?

Imitation and role modeling are learning approaches that do not rely on conscious awareness but do involve imaging. Gardner (1983) describes these approaches as traditionally superior in learning interpersonal and bodily-kinesthetic skills. Bandura's social learning theory (Swenson, 1980) is one educational model that has imitation and modeling as central ideas. Role modeling has been highly valued in nursing education for interpersonal and attitudinal learning, and it can be seen that this approach has a solid neurological basis.

In Hart's (1983) approach, modeling would be one of numerous experiences in which learners might be involved. A myriad of experiential activities are important. From multiple exposures to and experiences of caring behavior and from multiple explorations about caring, the brain naturally begins to form a pattern of integrated caring behavior.

SUMMARY

We can see that by transferring caring behaviors from previous experiences, by imitation of role models, and by multiple experiential activities, learners form and utilize schemata of caring. By finding ways to stimulate learners to think about the feeling of caring and to imagine caring for others, caring becomes a psychophysiological or psychokinesthetic experience. A broad aim or high-level purpose, that is, to care, to have interest in and concern for others, or union and separation toward growth could serve as an inner context that would automatically evoke associated networks of learned, integrated caring actions. The caregiver would not usually be aware of each separate action. These broad aims would organize procedural knowledge, or "know how," in the motor areas of the brain.

Let us return to Garfield's predicament. Can we help him walk again? Perhaps someone will call him in a friendly voice, someone whom he knows will give him a little chow and lots of stroking on his head. I suspect he would forget about his feet and just hurry over.

REFERENCES

Benner, P. (1984). *From novice to expert: Excellence and power in clinical nursing practice.* Menlo Park, CA: Addison-Wesley.

Benner, P., & Wrubel, J. (1988). *The primacy of caring: Stress and coping in health and illness.* Menlo Park, CA: Addison-Wesley.

Bobrow, D. G., & Norman, D. A. (1975). Some principles of memory schemata. In B. G. Bobrow & A. Collins (Eds.), *Representation and understanding: Studies in cognitive science* (pp. 131–149). New York: Academic Press.

Cohen, N. J., & Squire, L. R. (1980). Preserved learning and retention of pattern-analyzing skill in amnesia: Dissociation of knowing how and knowing that. *Science, 210,* 207–210.

Flannery, J., & Taylor, G. (1981). Toward integrating psyche and soma: Psycho-analysis and neurobiology. *Canadian Journal of Psychiatry, 26,* 15–23.

Gallwey, W. T. (1974). *The inner game of tennis.* New York: Bantam.

Gardner, H. (1983). *Frames of mind: The theory of multiple intelligences.* New York: Basic Books.

Gazzaniga, M. S. (1985). *The social brain: Discovering networks of the mind.* New York: Basic Books.

Gendron, D. (1988). *The expressive form of caring.* Toronto: University of Toronto, Faculty of Nursing, Perspectives in Caring, Monograph II.

Hart, L. A. (1975). *How the brain works.* New York: Basic Books.

Hart, L. A. (1983). *Human brain and human learning.* New York: Longman.

John, E. R. (1980). A neurophysiological model of purposive behavior. In R. F. Thompson, L. H. Hicks, & V. B. Shvyrkov (Eds.), *Neural mechanisms of goal-directed behavior and learning* (pp. 93–110). New York: Academic Press.

Pribram, K. (1971). *Languages of the brain.* Englewood Cliffs, NJ: Prentice-Hall.

Pribram, K. (1980). The place of pragmatics in the syntactic and semantic organization of language. In H. W. Dechert & M. Raupach (Eds.), *Temporal variables in speech* (pp. 13–20). The Hague: Moulton.

Rumelhart, D. (1980). Schemata: The building blocks of cognition. In R. J. Spiro, B. C. Bruce, & W. F. Brewer (Eds.), *Theoretical issues in reading comprehension* (pp. 33–55). Hillsdale, NJ: Erlbaum.

Schacter, D. L., & Moscovitch, M. (1984). Infants, amnesics, and dissociable memory systems. In M. Moscovitch (Ed.), *Infant memory: Its relation to normal and pathological memory in humans and animals* (pp. 173–216). New York: Plenum Press.

Squire, L. R. (1984). The neuropsychology of memory. In P. Marler & H. S. Terrace (Eds.), *The biology of learning* (pp. 667–685). Berlin: Springer-Verlag.

Swenson, L. C. (1980). *Theories of learning: Traditional perspectives / contemporary developments.* Belmont, CA: Wadsworth.

26

The Lived Experience of Nursing Education: A Phenomenological Study

Tommie P. Nelms

It has been called reconceptualization by curriculum theorists, it has been called curriculum revolution by Em Bevis, it has been called reform and renaissance by others—new notions of curriculum that focus on the individual and the context of the individual's existence. Ultimately within these reconceived notions of curriculum that espouse freedom, choice, existence, and transcendence in education, there is no curriculum until each individual reflects and creates personal meaning of the planned learnings. For these educators a curriculum only becomes a curriculum as it is experienced by the individual, creating meaning and releasing potential.

One of the courses that I took as a doctoral student was titled "Curriculum Leaders." My fellow classmates and I were to choose a curriculum leader, read everything the leader had published, contact him or her if alive, and prepare a paper and a presentation about our selection for the class. The leader that I chose was Maxine Greene. I found her work to be beautiful, powerful, and inspiring. When I contacted her by phone, she told me first that she did not consider herself a curriculum leader, but rather an educational philosopher who had

285

something to say about curriculum. I asked Dr. Greene about a brief autobiography that appears in *Curriculum Theorizing* (Pinar, 1975) which she called "that embarrassing biography" where she stated, "and I don't want to die before I read at least a tenth of what I want to read, before I learn something, before I really can say I understand what teaching is" (p. 298). When I asked her if she really believed that she hadn't learned anything, she said she would have to answer me from her existential background, her landscape, as it were. She said, "I am what I am not yet." She elaborated that we are always in the process of becoming. There is always something else to reach for and this is what we must know and impart as teachers.

It was Maxine Greene who started the spark of curriculum reconceptualization burning within me. From there I came to know and love three other reconceptualists: Dwayne Huebner, James Macdonald, and William Pinar. The ideas of these four formed the conceptual framework for my study of the lived experience of undergraduate nursing education.

The purpose of this study was to provide a theoretical base on which nursing education could incorporate the lived experience of nursing students into its curriculum through phenomenological methodology. Specific objectives were:

1. To incorporate one idea of the curriculum reconceptualized by systematically illuminating the "lived experience" of a group of persons experiencing nursing education and the meaningfulness of the experience in their lives.

2. To incorporate another idea of the curriculum reconceptualized by determining if there is what Pinar (1975) calls a "transbiographic" phenomenon of the lived experience of nursing education (a collective transpersonal realm of education).

3. Having gained this knowledge, to suggest ways in which reconceptualist ideas can be used to enhance the aims and purposes of nursing education.

In this study I interviewed 17 nursing students at Georgia State University in the three levels of the generic baccalaureate nursing program. My 11 years of nursing teaching experience at that time, the tacit knowledge that I possessed about the existences of nursing students, and my study of curriculum reconceptualization and phenomenology all led me to believe that the following interview questions would answer the research questions of this study.

Questions 1 and 2—What made you decide to become a nurse? What made you decide to come to Georgia State University to become a nurse?—were proposed to make the students comfortable as the interview began.

Question 3—What things have been the most meaningful to you as a nursing student? or What are the most positive things about your life as a nursing student?—was proposed because this information would give knowledge of the students' lived experiences, the meaningfulness of nursing education in their lives, and their existence along the journey. Although *meaning* is a concept that pervades the reconceptualized notion of curriculum, reconceptualist ideas, and phenomenological tradition, it was thought that students might have difficulty with the term *meaningful;* therefore, question 3 was rephrased for clarification.

Question 4—What things are less than positive, if not negative experiences, about being a nursing student?—was also proposed to help illuminate lived experience, meaning, and existence along the nursing education journey. The question was phrased this way because I did not want to predispose the students into sharing negative experiences if they experienced none. I do not believe that the concept of meaning as dealt with by reconceptualists and phenomenologists has a value connotation. However, common usage connotes a positive value to the term *meaningful.* Therefore, by proposing questions that connoted the sharing of both positive (question 3) and less than positive (question 4) aspects of nursing education, I hoped to obtain the broadest possible range of meanings in the lives of the students.

Question 5—What are some examples or some incidents when you feel really understood about what you are experiencing as a nursing student?—was proposed because the concept of feeling understood is associated with having one's existence or lived experience confirmed. The concept of perceived understanding by another is often the initial focus of phenomenological study (Omery, 1983).

Questions 6 and 7—Do you feel that you as a person with a life and roles outside of nursing are ever recognized? and Do you recognize the faculty as people outside their faculty role?—were proposed to see if temporality, biography, and multifaceted personhood were a part of the lived experience of nursing education and whether these concepts have meaning for nursing students.

Finally, question 8—Do you ever have experiences with either the content or the processes of nursing and learning to be a nurse that you would like to share? and Are you able to share your feelings about your experiences with others?—was asked to determine whether students are called on or given opportunity to verbalize their self-reflection as they live the process of becoming a nurse.

The phenomenological methodology allowed the individual lived experiences of the nursing students to be systematically illuminated. The commonalities of the students' experiences revealed a collective transbiographic phenomenon. The categories that emerged in the transpersonal realm of their experiences with individual anecdotes are presented here, along with the meaning of these experiences for future nursing curricula. These categories are not exclusive; the experiences overlap and interrelate. Before I illuminate the phenomenon, however, I would like to offer an apology to my co-researchers. Dwayne Huebner has said that since the beginning of time, philosophers, artists, poets, theologians, and the like have tried to capture the essence of human beings only to have it escape time and time again. Yet we in curriculum have the temerity to reduce the mystery, awe, and wonder of human beings to one term, "learner" (Huebner, 1975).

LIFE-PERVASIVE INTENSIVE COMMITMENT

The phenomenon of what it is to live the experience of a nursing student as illuminated in this study is that of a life-pervasive intensive commitment to a personal goal. It is an experience in which students feel a tremendous sense that there are almost insurmountable amounts of knowledge to be learned and mastered. Students made statements like: "the pressure—the constant pressure" and "I never thought it was so time-consuming and demanding." Students are continuously aware that the knowledge and skills to be mastered must be mastered according to certain criteria and within a certain time frame, and that any deviations will result in their dismissal from the program. And these students are always aware that dismissal from the program means waiting at least one full year before re-entering. This aspect of their experience, although serving as a motivator, also deters from the enjoyment of the pursuit of a personal commitment made and intended by the student.

Students talked about never really being able to relax during the quarter, as if a dark cloud of nursing was hanging over them at all times because of the work they had to do. As one student said, "When I'm not studying nursing, I feel guilty. I cannot sit down and read a magazine because I should be reading my nursing book." Many students discussed having no social life or no time to themselves. Regarding their social lives, they said such things as: "I feel my social growth has been

stifled as a single person," "People always said that college was supposed to be the best years of your life, but I don't think so," and "All the
study time leaves no time for a social life."

This time-consuming, intense nature of nursing education was discussed by all students as the least positive aspect of their lived experience. Certainly some of this aspect of nursing education is outside the
control of the nursing education system. A tremendous knowledge base
must be learned by nursing students and this knowledge base is growing
all the time. There are also competencies that must be mastered with
exact precision. Faculty members, as the designers and administrators
of nursing curricula, can neither deny these facts nor require less of
nursing graduates. Faculty can, however, remain aware that nursing
education is very intensive, stressful, and time-consuming in the lives
of the students. Students talked about expecting faculty to be aware of
their lived experience in this regard or expecting faculty to acknowledge an awareness of this nature of nursing education and their disap-
pointment when such awareness was not forthcoming. As one student
stated, "I felt that there were not enough faculty to go to, to ease
tension, not to make it easier, but just to listen." Another student said,
"It's great when some faculty act like they still remember what it was
like to be a student. I don't know why they all can't be that way; they all
went to nursing school, too!"

A strong theme that emerged in this category was that life is put on
hold while persons pursue nursing education. Opposition to this theme
is one that is addressed throughout the work of curriculum reconceptualists. Huebner's (1975) ethical rationality sets forth the following
ideas: educational activity is life, life's meanings are witnessed and lived
in the classroom. Within education it is the human situation, the encounter of teacher to student, that is of utmost importance. This encounter is the essence of life. For Huebner the content to be taught is simply
the arena of human confrontation. A shift in focus within nursing education from the content and skills to be mastered to a focus on the lives
involved in these encounters could help students come to believe that
life doesn't stop when nursing education begins.

THE MEANING OF CLINICAL

Students told me unanimously that the single most meaningful aspect of
their lived experiences was their clinical experiences. They said such
things as: "Clinical is where I get my good feelings about myself and my

patients," "Clinical is where I can touch other people's lives," "Clinical is what tells me that I am doing the right thing with my life." Clinical for these students was transcendence—a time and space to transcend the hard work and long hours of pre-planning, class, and studying to focus in that space and time on caring for their patients and creating themselves as nurses. One student said to me, "If I never graduate or become an RN, the clinical experiences that I have had and the good feelings I have had about myself and the lives that I have touched, it was accomplished. What I wanted to do was accomplished." I find this to be a powerful existential statement of this student's lived experience as a nursing student.

The meaningfulness of clinical for these students emerged on two levels. One is that the clinical experiences give meaning to these students' lives as they interacted with and helped other people and also in that it was within the context of their clinical experiences that they developed and began to feel good about their ability to perform competently as nurses. That these students already saw clinical and caring as the core of nursing was very affirming for me as a nursing educator who would like us to reconceive our notions of curriculum. In all our years of trying to fit nursing curricula into the behaviorist rationale, the one thing that never quite fit was clinical. Yes, we planned for it and wrote objectives for it and even tried to measure and grade it, but we always accepted that on some level it would be serendipitous, as the artist Reinhold Marxhausen has said, "the possibility of happy, chance discovery."

Time is precious in nursing education programs. Transcending our old beliefs about how persons come to possess knowledge and conceiving new modes of nursing curricula that enhance the kinds of knowledge acquired through clinical practice and clinical praxis would be time well spent for nurse educators. We must rethink our traditional uses of class time and our enslavement to old teaching methods—such as the lecture—that perpetuate power struggles in nursing education.

PERSONAL KNOWLEDGE EXPERIENCES

I specifically asked students if they ever had experiences with the content of nursing when they knew that it had really become their knowledge; when they might say to themselves, "Hey, this is my knowledge now, I know this!" I asked the question because I believe what Polanyi (1958) contends, that all knowledge is personal knowledge because there is nothing known that isn't known by a person. All these students recounted that they did have these experiences, saying things such as, "Yeah, it happens all the time. I always feel excited when I understand something, especially when something seemed like it was so stupid to learn to start with—like why am I learning this? And then you see it in action. Yeah, it's real good" and "It has been happening a lot this quarter. I'm saying to myself, gosh, I can do this!" Another student stated, "Yeah, definitely, because this is what I have been striving for this whole time, to be somebody. I put a lot of value in education and the college degree itself. It means a lot to me and who I am and how people perceive me. So that definitely makes me feel good when I'm able to convey my knowledge." Other students shared that they did have these experiences and that they made them feel good. One student shared that when she had such experiences, she breathed a "sigh of relief" and said to herself, "I am in the right profession. It happened on clinical last week, everything seemed to click. It felt great and I was so relieved."

On establishing that the students did, in fact, have such experiences when nursing knowledge became their personal knowledge, I then asked if they shared these experiences and, if so, with whom. The majority said they did share such experiences, most often with classmate/friends, family, and instructors. One student said, "I share with others (classmates) and I hope they will share with me. It's real exciting!" Others talked of sharing these experiences with their mothers or their boyfriends. Student responses were mixed regarding sharing these experiences with faculty. One student said, "I share with my instructor if they are directly involved. Instructors love it! They like knowing that they are doing their job, and they like knowing that you are learning." But another said, "I think, oh this is great, but I don't share it with instructors because I think they are not interested."

Students were then asked if they felt that they were encouraged to share such experiences and whether it would benefit their lives or this program if more sharing were done. Most agreed that they weren't encouraged to share their personal knowledge experiences and, if they ever were, it was only from a few faculty and in very limited situations. Some of their responses were: "There aren't enough opportunities; you forget good experiences before you get together again," "If there was a forum for that kind of thing I would share, but we aren't asked and I don't volunteer," "Sharing this would make the program better, but I wouldn't want to share, although I am happy in myself that it happens."

The fact that these students have these personal knowledge experiences, the fact that these experiences are meaningful to their lives, and the fact that they share these experiences with friends, family, and in-structors is highly significant. However, as these students revealed, recognizing these experiences and sharing these experiences is not an integral part of their nursing education. Yet these are the kinds of experiences that would broaden the definition of curriculum. They are the kinds of experiences that are needed in nursing education programs that accept that curriculum is not curriculum until its meaningfulness is revealed in the lives of those experiencing it.

These students reveal that their nursing curriculum stops short of recognizing or requiring of them the meaningfulness of nursing knowledge and skills in their lives. Their curriculum stops at acquisition of nursing knowledge and skills. Again, it is positive that some students believe that faculty like hearing of their personal knowledge experiences and recognize that this confirms for faculty that they are "doing their jobs." Yet it is less than positive that others perceive that their instructors would not even be interested in these experiences in their lives.

SUPPORT SYSTEMS

Another theme that emerged as very meaningful to the lived experiences of these students was their support systems along this educational journey. The groups mentioned most often were fellow classmates, "a couple of" instructors, and some nurses at the hospital, in that order.

Understandably, these students reported that their nursing classmates were now their best friends and that those friendships offered them their strongest sources of support. Several students talked about seeking out those persons in the class who, because of similar life situations, could offer them understanding and support. One student talked about the fact that the younger, single students tended to group together, while the married students with families did the same. Several students talked about how quickly and strongly they had become "bonded" to their classmates, now their friends, in nursing, something that had not happened to them in other classes or educational programs.

One student who had recently completed a degree in political science at Georgia State University said that she had had classes with many of the same people consistently in her political science studies but had never come to know them as well or as closely as her nursing classmates. When asked why she thought this was so, she said it was because in political science there wasn't the "do or die—them against us" attitude that she had experienced in nursing, and it was that attitude that nursing students experienced in their lives and understood in the lives of others. Another student expressed it this way, "We all have a kind of camaraderie or a feeling that we're all toughing it out together." Another student said, "Maybe it is selfish, but I get great satisfaction just sitting back quietly and listening to other students talk, hearing them express the same things that I've been experiencing, just knowing that I'm not the only one that feels this way."

Again students valued greatly the support that they received from faculty members and staff nurses, but all were surprised at how few of these two groups were genuinely supportive of their lived experience, especially since both these groups had at one time experienced nursing education themselves. These students really liked it when faculty and staff nurses told them of their errors or experiences in nursing school. One student said she felt relieved and hopeful when told of an error made in nursing school by a staff nurse. As she stated, "Wow, if she's this smart now, then there's hope for me!"

Although a great source of support, these students report that their families and their friends outside nursing education don't really understand what their lives are like as nursing students. This is one factor that brings them so close to their fellow classmates, because no one on the "outside," so to speak, can ever really understand the intensity of pursuing nursing education.

As nursing educators we need to find ways to capitalize on this strong sense of support that students enjoy from each other. Learning activities could be developed that use this sense of support to enhance knowledge acquisition in an air of camaraderie instead of an air of competition. This sense of being responsible for one's own learning as well as that of one's classmates could transfer into clinical practice where nurses would willingly share their knowledge in a caring way with others, rather than selfishly withholding their knowledge from peers and patients.

FEELINGS ABOUT SELF

This category had a very temporal nature. Students' feelings about self began to emerge when asked about their reasons for pursuing nursing education. These students shared great knowledge gained through self-reflection about why they were seeking to become a nurse. They spoke of recognizing their desires to interact in certain ways with other human beings or their beliefs that nurses act in certain ways and must know certain things that they believe they would be suited to, based on their recognition of who they were and what they believed their capabilities to be. They spoke of their consciousness of their personality traits and of how some of these traits developed in their lives. They spoke of these traits as being those that they believe a nurse must have and their goal now to have their personality traits merge with those they believe are important in nursing, as they emerge as the person that they are, who becomes a nurse.

They spoke of perceiving experiences in their pasts that did not gibe with their perceptions of who they were and what they wanted to do with their lives. Two students spoke of not wanting to sit in a microbiology lab all day without ever really knowing the person whose lab test results they were observing. One student with a very successful career in retail sales spoke of not getting enough of what she called the feeling of "fortunateness" in her life, while another student with a degree in music performance recognized that such a degree would not bring her the things in her life that she believed a nursing degree would.

The most positive aspects of these students' lives in nursing education, second only to their clinical experiences, were their feelings about themselves. They shared such achievements in this category as: "having a goal and purpose to my life, as opposed to waiting tables, and the reaction I get from people when I say I'm in nursing school"; "personal growth, seeing something from beginning to end and especially now that I am in my thirties"; "the feeling of accomplishment of having gone this far. I don't feel pressure from my parents or the faculty. I've done it myself. I've motivated myself. I've never stuck with anything this long"; and "knowing that each quarter brings me closer to my personal goals."

Other students talked about the feeling of accomplishment at fitting nursing education into their already full lives as mothers, wives, boyfriends, church members, and employees. They talked about their feelings about the knowledge they were gaining and how that knowledge affected other areas of their lives. Things that they felt were meaningful were: "the knowledge that I have gained—so much in such a short time, about nursing, about people, about myself," "having knowledge of nursing carry over into my home life; being able to care for my grandmother," and "being competent in the caregiver role and dealing with patients has given me confidence for dealing with situations in my life outside of nursing; it has made me more assertive, given me confidence and helped my self-esteem." Becoming more accepting of others was meaningful to another student. As she stated, "Nursing has made me more accepting of others. I have learned to like someone that I couldn't stand at first. I realize she has needs too. This is one of my biggest influences of nursing school."

The illumination of the lived experiences of these students reveals that they are temporal beings-in-the-world who experience much self-reflection to create the meanings that nursing education holds for their lives: past, present, and future. Yet these students convey that the curriculum provides them little opportunity to verbalize the self-reflection that they experience as they live the process of becoming a nurse. Maxine Greene (1974) conceives of curriculum as possibility, possibility for all individuals. As she states, "personally significant and liberating learning can only take place when the learner is able to articulate and make explicit what is involved as 'meaning emerges,' the meaning constituted through heightened consciousness" (Greene, 1974, p. 73). As nursing educators we must give students structured opportunities to share the meanings that all aspects of nursing education create in their lives. These opportunities need to be viewed and valued as valid educational activities just as lectures, skills practice, and clinical experiences are.

IDEAL TEACHER

The lived experience of these students reveals that they expect many things of those that teach them. Whether they experience it or not, students expect to be recognized as a person and a fellow human being, just as they expect to be allowed to see the personhood of the instructor. Their responses were mixed on this issue. As some students stated: "We are a small class, so we do more talking about personal things" and "They see us as people but expect us to have nursing as the priority in our lives; boyfriends come after nursing care plans and drug cards." Another student was very philosophical about this issue, as he stated, "Some faculty are more personable than others. One instructor, I won't mention any names, said that she didn't want to be anyone's friend. She wanted to keep it on a professional basis because she said you get in trouble when you do that."

These students expect recognition of the amount of knowledge to be acquired and mastered. They expect some effort on the part of the teacher to learn from them how their learning is progressing. They expect that those teaching them are competent, caring, and supportive. They expect that their teachers value the importance of nursing knowledge and competency but never more than they value them as a person. They expect to be treated as adults who have prior knowledge of many things, but who now are willing to accept the responsibility for acquiring nursing knowledge. They expect that those teaching them will stand before them striving to be centered, authentic persons who in turn strive to look for the center of those they encounter; an I-thou encountering each other.

It is a lived experience in which these students recognize that the core of education is the one-to-one, student-to-teacher encounter, as evidenced by the fact that in most cases the value of any learning experience was directly related to the personality of those who teach them and their one-to-one interaction with that person.

James Macdonald (1981) saw as part of a total curriculum plan the quality of lived experience in the relationships of subject to subject, persons to society, and persons to persons. He espoused the concepts of centering and authenticity for both teachers and students within the framework of curriculum. He set forth that the ultimate question to be answered by curriculum planners in any educational setting should be, How shall we live together?

As planners of nursing curricula, we have struggled with our subject to subject relationships and our nursing profession to society relationships, but we have not often addressed the question of how we shall live together in our person-to-person relationships within schools of nursing.

A quote that I encountered in my study of curriculum reconceptualization changed my life because it has made me see things in ways I had not seen before and has made me examine the assumptions on which I live my life. In it James Macdonald calls us to transcend our focus on individualization and recognize our connectedness to all other human beings:

> The person is valued because of what he shares in common with all persons: the human condition. Each person strives to create meaning out of his existence in the world and attempts to gain freedom from crippling fear, anxiety, and guilt. Each person shares the common fate of mortality and possesses the potential for expressing joy, awe and wonder. The awareness that all we know with certainty is that we are here and that there are others like us, characterizes the human condition and makes the person of value. Thus it is not the uniqueness of the individual in terms of this personal perceptions, idiosyncratic needs, desires, and motives that makes him of value; it is his common status (Burke, 1985, p. 95).

I believe that raising the nursing education consciousness to reconceptualist ideas and ideals and incorporating their notions of curriculum into the nursing education system and the nursing care system are but modes of entry into relationships between fellow human beings who experience a common human condition. The reconceptualization of curriculum is a caring, ethical undertaking that must be accomplished by nurse educators who believe that the creation of more just nursing education is our part of making a more just public world. We can do no less.

REFERENCES

Burke, M. M. (Fall, 1985). The personal and professional journey of James B. Macdonald. *Journal of Curriculum Theorizing, 6*(3), 84–119.

Greene, M. (1974). Cognition, consciousness, and curriculum. In W. Pinar (Ed.), *Heightened consciousness, cultural revolution, and curriculum theory* (pp. 69–84). Berkeley, CA: McCutchan.

Huebner, D. (1975). Curricular language and classroom meanings. In W. Pinar (Ed.), *Curriculum theorizing: The reconceptualists* (pp. 217–236). Berkeley, CA: McCutchan.

Macdonald, J. B. (1981). Curriculum, consciousness and social change. *Journal of Curriculum Theorizing, 3*(1), 143–153.

Omery, A. (1983). Phenomenology: A method for nursing research. *Advances in Nursing Science, 5*(2), 49–63.

Pinar, W. (1975). Currere: Toward reconceptualization. In W. Pinar (Ed.), *Curriculum theorizing: The reconceptualists* (pp. 396–414). Berkeley, CA: McCutchan.